DIET·FREE DIVA

5 Steps to Freedom With Food-Body-Self on Your Trusted and Sustainable Terms

TRACY L. DESJARDINS, IAHC

THE DIET-FREE DIVA

5 Steps to Freedom With Food-Body-Self on Your Trusted and Sustainable Terms

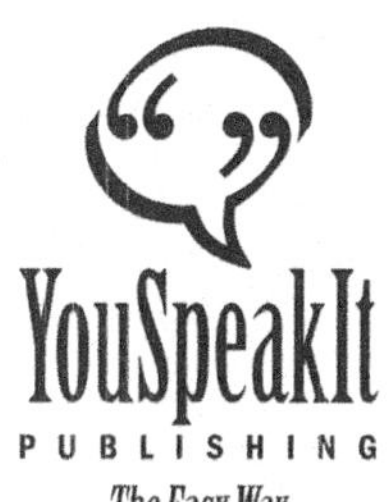

ISBN: 978-0-9753668-4-4

To amazing women like you, who are fed up with dieting, restricting, obsessing, and seeking a sustainable solution to their struggles with food, body, and self.

Praise For *The Diet-Free Diva*

"*The Diet-Free Diva* provides a deep healing pathway out of the weight loss wars and helps women find their own answers with eating challenges that they can live with forever."

— Mike Collins, Founder of SugarAddiction.com, Leader of the Sugar Addiction & Detox Community, Sugar Addiction Peer Recovery, and The Quit Sugar Summit

"I laughed, cried, highlighted countless quotes, and shouted 'yes' all the way through *The Diet-Free Diva!* Tracy's friendly, girl-next-door demeanor makes women feel connected, understood, and inspired to begin taking steps towards believing that we can find our own solutions to healing our body-mind-food relationship. *The Diet-Free Diva* is essential for any woman fed up by the confusion: this book and Tracy are the real deal!"

— Lisa Michaud, Entrepreneur, Success Coach, Speaker, and Host of the Goalden Girls Podcast

"This book is written from the heart. It shares the bold truths about the negative ramifications of dieting, to empower its readers to embrace their joy, and create a movement towards healing from emotional eating challenges."

— Robert Notter, Marketing & Mindset Success Coach

"*The Diet-Free Diva* is an inspiration for any woman who is living a similar battle with yo-yo dieting and negative self-talk and only wants truth."

— Jenn Edden, Founder of The Sugar Freedom Method
and Author of *Woman Unleashed*

"Tracy's unapologetic stance on the problems with dieting culture in this book is a refreshing take on how we can truly take back our lives, find out what truly nourishes us on every level, and discover how food is our friend that helps us shed unwanted pounds naturally."

— Mark Sasscer, Founder of LeadQuest Consulting, Inc.,
World-Class Business Leader, and Author

"In *The Diet-Free Diva*, Tracy eliminates the needless guilt that many feel in regards to food and inspires readers to begin taking steps towards believing that we can find our own solutions to our eating concerns."

— Jenn Hamilton, DPT, CPT, Physical Therapist,
and Business Owner

"When you're looking to change your relationship with food, you can't beat a guide like Tracy who walks the talk every day!"

— Dan DeFigio, Author of
Beating Sugar Addiction For Dummies

"Tracy is soul medicine that EVERY woman needs in their life. *The Diet-Free Diva* shines a big beautiful spotlight on everything we are not looking at... the honest truth."

— Errin Smith, Founder and Host, What We Crave: The Emotional Eating Summit

"This book tells the truth about how to recover from decades of fighting ourselves to finally release the extra weight."

— Keith Leon S., 7x Award-Winning 9x International Bestselling Author and Publisher

"*The Diet-Free Diva* is one of the best, no-nonsense, truth be told books for exposing the negative ramifications of dieting and offers an effective, groundbreaking program for healing from emotional eating challenges."

— Kathy Robbins, LICSW, PCC, SRC, Psychotherapist and Life Coach

"Tracy Desjardins has created a wonderful book that's all about finding real and lasting freedom with food and body. You'll discover important insights, helpful tools and a wealth of information and wisdom to help you on your own unique journey. This book is written in a style that's honest, wise, and easy to follow. Highly recommended!"

— Marc David, Author and Founder of the Institute for the Psychology of Eating

"Tracy writes straight from the heart with enthusiasm, energy and passion. With candor and warmth, she details her personal battles with the weight-loss lies we have all been sold for decades. The strategies Tracy puts forward are sustainable, holistic and health-affirming. If you are exhausted by punishing workouts and unrealistic diets, you need to read *The Diet-Free Diva*."

— Antonia Ryan, Author of
The 10 Day Binge Eating Detox Plan,
Mindfulness for Binge Eating, and
Letting Go Of Overeating

Contents

Acknowledgments

I thank God for giving me the courage to write this book and for the lifelong challenges I faced in my personal food battleground. His timing taught me the lessons I needed to learn in order to help me understand at a deep level food and body challenges so that I can be of service to other women who are struggling.

To Gary, Emily, and Jackson: Thank you for being the wind beneath my wings in ways that I cannot describe. I continue to be humbled by your love, support, and authentic hearts. I am forever grateful to be your wife and mother.

To my parents, Mike and Pat: Thank you for your unending love and believing in my potential.

To Jackson Desjardins, my son who is my ultimate example of resilient sunshine, positivity, and courage: Thank you for being unapologetically *you* at all times and inspiring me to break out of my fears. You make the world a better place. Never change.

To Danielle Daem and Lisa Michaud: For being the diva-forces that pulled me out of hiding and taught me what tools I need to fly outside of my comfort zone: I am forever grateful for your heartfelt inspiration.

Thank you to Mike Collins, the Sugar Detox Support Group, and the Quit Sugar Summit for being my launching pad for personal healing and ongoing support—*onward!*

To Marc David and Julie M. Simon: Thank you for teaching about emotional eating and showing me a healing pathway that literally saved my life.

To all my wonderful clients I have the grace of working with over the last three-plus decades: Thank you for the opportunity to serve you and to create fitness and wellness magic with movement and connection together.

Thank you to the wonderful staff at YouSpeakIt Publishing, especially Rona Gofstein and Heather Taylor, for their patient coaching and helping me to believe that my creative voice is valid and needed in this world.

A Note From the Author

I wrote this book for you, girlfriends, who are ready and wanting answers to your unwanted eating concerns.

You are tired of the fight with food, finding the right diet, and putting your dreams and potential on hold until you lose the weight and get yourself on track. I understand you because I lived this battle most of my life. I promise you that there is a better way. I invite you to be open and curious to a new perspective that you may have never considered.

There is a pathway for you out of this inner, personal war. You are not alone, and this war is not your fault. Thank you for giving me this opportunity to share my personal, raw truth and vulnerability with you. My hopes are that, together, we make a common connection where *you* feel validated, affirmed, inspired, and empowered to believe you can find your way out of destructive dieting and emotional eating challenges and finally find peace with food, body, and self in a manner that sustains and supports you.

Together, we will create a movement toward health and healing *on your terms* and discover how to rock your inner Diva who is held captive in your private war with food. Together, we form a movement toward common sense and take back your power to live your best life as who you are meant to be.

Tracy Desjardins

Introduction

Hello, my friend! When you see or hear the word *diet*, do you cringe as I do?

Do you associate diets with suffering, pain, failure, and fighting?

Are you confused by the constantly changing dieting plans that contradict each other and only make us crazy?

Then you and I are going to become pals. This book is dedicated to *you*, the smart woman who is sick and tired of this *diet* concept in general. You want real solutions for your challenges with food, body, and self. You can harness your life as your *Best Diva Self*—the self who lives a life of purpose and passion without the constant distractions of fighting yourself over food.

My name is Tracy Desjardins, and I am a fitness professional of more than thirty years. I chose to shift my concentration from exercise to holistic wellness coaching for women because I had become entirely fed up with the façade and lies of the diet industry in which I lived and battled on a deep, personal level for decades. I tried to compensate for my problems with food by exercising my ass off.

I am here to *shout from the rooftops!* that this does not work; neither do diets and the act of dieting. Dieting is on the spectrum of *eating restriction*. In other words, you may not think you are a dieter, per se, but if you are restricting your food intake and depriving yourself, going crazy from starting over when you fail at your *plan*, then you are dieting, my friend.

Exercise is just one component of living one's best life. I am deliberately becoming part of a movement toward truth and healing from a common challenge in the fitness industry—hardworking people fighting with exercise and diets to lose weight and change their bodies. That was my personal battle for more than thirty-five years.

I chased a specific body image, a number on the scale, and I believed that I could out-exercise poor eating habits to achieve success. *Success* meant slimming down to societal standards and feeling validated and worthy as a person, especially as a fitness professional who was supposed to be the billboard of inspiration and have the perfect body and all the answers. I hid behind my diet-driven, binge-eating shame and interior war for decades.

Many people like me spend years, if not decades, fighting themselves and constantly starting over with a new diet plan and a demanding exercise regimen that feels punishing. This becomes a vicious cycle of hope and defeat. It is truly exhausting on every level—physical, emotional, mental, and spiritual. Exercise complements a holistic lifestyle in which food is a nurturing, loving friend, not an enemy. Many women have this backward, as I did for decades.

My work as a holistic health coach focuses on helping women find healing from destructive dieting, cultivating a path of personal excellence with food, body, and self on their unique terms that will sustain them for life.

There is no other way. This is smart healing.

In this book, I share my battle. I struggled for acceptance according to society's standards. After decades of trial and tribulation, I returned to myself by collecting strategic tools in my healing toolbox. I stopped fighting myself. I discovered freedom when I stopped dieting and began thinking, feeling, and *being*.

What constitutes a *Diet* and what is *Dieting?*

According to several dictionaries, a *diet* is a chosen set of foods that an individual consumes, with certain inclusions and restrictions, with an anticipated outcome of positive, healthy change—typically weight loss or change of body size. Another definition includes the "selection of food is especially as designed or prescribed to improve a person's physical condition or to prevent or treat a disease."[1]

Is dieting a successful strategy for maintaining health?

1 dictionary.com

Diets as prescribed by healthcare professionals for individualized health concerns, for instance, for type 2 diabetes or heart disease, are of course necessary and, in some cases, can be lifesaving. However, diets that are designed *for the goal of weight loss only* are of polarized debate.

Research shows that 80–95 percent of dieters regain weight after pushing through an unsustainable, overly restrictive diet plan.[2] That surely sounds like failure.

In this book, I share my *5 Steps to Find Freedom With Food-Body-Self* that lovingly guide you out of the war with dieting and fighting yourself with food. I introduce tools for finding a healing pathway out of diets and restrictions and toward the most precious gifts of all: trusting yourself with food and finding sustainable peace within yourself, perhaps for the first time ever. What awaits is what I call *your Best Diva Self*—the *you* the world needs you to be.

Onward!

2 "Why People Diet, Lose Weight and Gain It All Back." 2019. health.clevelandclinic.org

CHAPTER ONE

Your Food Story

DEEP DIVE! YOUR PERSONAL HISTORY WITH FOOD

Have you ever wondered what the story is of your relationship with food?

The journey from infancy until now is a magnificent collection of powerful and secret messages of who you are as an eater. Food is a symbol: to some, a friend; to others, an enemy. It takes courage to consider there may be hope for food freedom beyond popular diet programs and all the gimmicks and supplements.

Current data indicate that the failure rate of diets is 95 percent.[3] I like to translate this into 95 percent of all diets fail *us*. The $72 billion diet industry grabs us at our vulnerable lows and hijacks our common sense to sell us the *perfect diet program* for weight loss. The genius marketing photos and

---

3 "The $72 Billion Weight Loss & Diet Control Market in the United States, 2019–2023." Feb. 2019. businesswire.com

advertisements lure us into believing our bodies and lives will transform to perfection, magically, with their diet.

The diet industry generates profits at the price of our hearts and souls. We get excited, buy into the diet, and when we *mess up*, we rebel, turn back to misusing food, and end up flat on our faces in shame, self-loathing, and feelings of failure and despair—until the next diet sells us the same false hopes. I've lost count of how many times, over thirty-five years, I fell for this destructive cycle.

Friend, if you are nodding your head here, you are not alone.

My personal food story took a very bumpy road. I was a free-spirited, happy child who was blissfully chubby. I had a great sense of humor and loved all things food—especially sugary junk foods and desserts because they just made me happy.

As I grew and life became complicated, I began *using* sugar in excessive quantities for immediate relief from whatever made me feel uncomfortable. Sugar was becoming my go-to best friend, my unconditional safety zone, and my therapist, all at the same time. I didn't realize it consciously.

This secret shame developed into a beast, starting in 1982 when I was around age twelve. I sold my soul in a desperate attempt to fix my body. I believed that my chubby self was unacceptable, I was embarrassing, and I was not good enough to fit in. I relied on my fighter instincts and began dieting and restricting food with the intent to *fix* myself.

As a result, my relationship with food, my body, and myself turned in a toxic, drama-filled battleground from within. My happy, free spirit that I once trusted went dormant. I developed a binge-eating problem in my early teens from every restricted and failed diet attempt. This plagued me for decades. I formed an invisible mask I wore to project the falsity that my life and I were awesome. But inside, I was hurting and privately fighting myself through restrictive dieting, bingeing, and starting over Monday morning more times that I can even count.

Diets promote a weight re-*gain* problem, not a weight *loss* solution. Truth be told here, diets *do* work, but only *if* the associated rules are followed precisely with a level of fierce, ongoing commitment that most rational people cannot fully embrace. I have personally experienced many weight-loss successes doing exactly that—spending tons of money and tons of time and tons of mental energy working the plan to extremes, focusing on a goal weight, pushing and fighting my way with the required plan, until weigh-in day. I would see my magic number of success on the dreaded scale, then lose interest, have no idea how to live with such restrictions, and gain every pound back plus more, at the high price of my self-respect.

Your Story Is Unique

Everyone is born into this world with an understanding that food, typically from Mother, brings instant comfort and love and safety. We learn to use food to celebrate and to satisfy many different emotions. Everyone has a food story, starting at infancy.

Our story and relationship with food is a fascinating collection of messages regarding who we are as an eater, and ultimately, a cultivation of our intimate relationship with our mind, body, and spirit. It is often a symbolic representation of how we relate to ourselves.

Our relationship with food is often an expression of how we are living our life. This reality is rarely explained in the diet phenomenon. It is an essential element of the human spirit. Eating is an experience that serves us with messages and clues as to how we are showing up in this thing called *Life*. Your journey and food story as an eater up till now offer insight on what is calling for our attention from within.

Your Story Is Valid

A common belief we share is:

food = instant comfort = pleasure

For most of us, our foundational conditioning begins in infancy, when we build understanding that nursing or feeding is a reliable source love, comfort, and safety. From our very first days out of the womb, we discover this:

1. Feel bad, cry

2. Be held and nurse or drink formula

3. Feel better *instantly*

As a child in the 1970s, I began soothing my uncomfortable emotions with sweets—cookies, candy, cake, ice cream, and so on. I noticed it delivered instant relief and consistently provided an escape. Without realizing it, I developed an abusive reliance on sugary foods. As a result, I became an overweight child.

Even though I was a free spirit, made tons of friends, and had a big personality, this practice of secret pig-outs felt shameful. I was a clever food-sneaker-in-training from an early age, and I was embarrassed by it. I could not seem to control it. I believed no one else in the world shared this problem. My expanding body was evidence of my problem with eating. This is my early food story.

Did you grow up with the concept: *Clean your plate because there are starving kids in third world countries?*

Or maybe you were forced to sit in torture at the table until you finished your veggies?

My husband is still haunted by that one! What if you were overly controlled by forced small portions? Or, you had to fight your siblings for the last cookie or bag of chips. Maybe as an adult, you find yourself rebelling from this control and eating as much as you want because now you can.

Are you like me, and remember the inner rebel raging when compared to thin and pretty girls?

Your unique food story is your truth and deserves to be respected and validated. We pick up messages and clues about food and eating throughout our lives. They show up for specific reasons and callings.

My subconscious security blanket became automatic, echoing that lesson learned in infancy: *Feel bad—eat food—feel better*. Many of us were taught to be tough and to ignore our feelings and emotions. This overwhelming burden can create a powerful, self-destructive habit of using food as a quick fix to escape from, cope with, and numb the pain of life's problems.

My friend, if this resonates with you, please know that your story is worthy, meaningful, and *valid*. Extend this understanding to yourself with compassion—not criticism, nor shame, nor judgment. It is an initial step in healing your relationship with food, body, and self.

Your Story Holds Clues

With my early habitual sugar binges to manage my emotions, the accompanying weight gain and inner toxic critical dialogue grew like a forest fire. In retrospect, these were clues that something was off in my life, but at the time, I did not recognize them. I could not get a handle on my overeating. I spent decades, after turning twelve in 1982, fighting myself with diets and restrictions. I went on a relentless quest to achieve my ideal weight, so that I could have the assurance of being worthy and loveable by the world. Something was calling out to me.

What was I missing?

What wasn't there *enough of* in my life that caused me to run and hide under sugar binges?

Allow me to emphasize here that the actual food is only one small clue of many. My food story continually presented me with personal struggles and challenges that demanded attention.

What was wrong with me?!

- What did I not understand?
- Why was I eating so much?
- Why did it seem like no one else had my problem?

My dysfunctional relationship with food revealed brilliantly what was missing in my heart and soul, but this did not reveal itself to me until decades later. The question of what is missing is an unconscious part of your story, and it is really not your fault when the dinner table becomes a battleground, or you've locked yourself in a food prison. This evolving problem of abusing food to cope with life can feel like your runaway train that surges out of control—a force that desperately needs to be turned around for rescue.

We have been taught by the diet industry that there is *good food* and *bad food*. This translates into the toxic mindset of equating what we eat to our integrity. When we eat good food, we are *being good*, and when we eat bad food, we are *being bad*. Follow these simple rules, and we are successful. Break the rules, and we are failures.

Research shows that some girls begin dieting as early as *ages seven to nine*.[4] In my quest to fit in, or be successful in society, I bought in to the dieting culture and failed over and over. I believed that if I achieved my goal weight as presented on charts, I would be accepted, loved, and *worthy* of having a place in this world.

This book is written especially for you who are tired of battling restrictive dieting and eating plans, binge eating, and starting over. If you desire the answer to why the struggle continues and to finally find a way out that is result-oriented and sustainable, read on!

RELATIONSHIP WITH APPETITE

Appetite is a hunger within—not just for food, but also for a vast spectrum of needs that call out to be filled. Appetite can refer to an inner drive for something awesome that we want in our lives. If channeled lovingly with proper inquiry, this

4 Abramovitz, Beth and Leann Birch. "Five-year-old girls' ideas about dieting are predicted by their mothers' dieting." DOI: 10.1016/S0002-8223(00)00339-4

appetite can reveal a beacon for the healing you deduce from your food story clues.

Dieting promotes a fear of hunger and appetite, which toxifies our natural-born instincts for survival and fulfillment. Feeling hunger can be misconstrued as *bad* or scary, and restricting or depriving oneself can be interpreted as being *good* or strong-willed and worthy of respect.

Instincts and Emotions

As mentioned before, when we are infants, we learn our needs have a better chance of being met if we make noise when something isn't right. Typically, someone hears our cry and answers our need. As we progress through life, we take this instinct with us and develop a subconscious language of instant gratification. We want what we want *right now* without mindful consideration.

When I felt a sugar binge coming on, it felt deep inside as though I had a kicking and screaming brat in my head who demanded what she wanted *now!* I had no skills of self-awareness, self-regulation, nor—*heaven forbid!*—self-compassion to sit with my feelings and know what I really needed, rather than excessive junk food that made me feel warm and fuzzy immediately, then sick, and ashamed.

Diet culture and drama fuel emotional binge eating by selling us on toxic programming that promotes a personal food rebellion. Dieting fuels toxicities like perfectionism and black-or-white thinking. Dieting robs us of our self-trust, respect, and dignity. In my decades of dieting, I never remember a diet program that explained the feelings and emotions of hunger. What results is the yo-yo effect of food- and rule-driven inner wars driven by instant gratification and sustained by the compulsion to feed our inner rebel.

It is time to learn to channel our natural-born food instincts and to understand the power of reining in the quest for instant gratification.

Dieting sells an approach founded in logic: If you do this and that, then you will lose weight. Weigh, measure, count, repeat. We all know these steps. Simple, right? We know what we should eat, but we don't know why we fail at consistently choosing well. This is because diets fail to address the emotional components of food and appetite. They only address rules, restriction, deprivation, and fighting oneself with the lone weapon of willpower.

Logic and emotion are completely different and are incompatible. Logic as it relates to dieting is also lacking in concepts that are sustainable. They are short-term, quick fixes. My guess is that you, dear reader, are *sick* of quick fixes that do not work.

We are emotionally driven humans with unique feelings and appetites. Any attempt to bypass or minimize the emotional components of eating and appetite will always end in disaster. We cannot *fight* our way toward healing our relationship with food. We will only heal when we meet ourselves with self-love and compassion. For most of us, this involves learning a whole new set of skills, but the good news is it can be done—and *you* can do it.

If you've come from a dieting background, approaching weight change from a place of love and acceptance seems odd. Diets do not teach love and compassion. Why not? There is no profit in it, friends. Love and compassion do not make money and cannot be purchased. They come from your heart, and they are free.

Food and Love

We catch on quickly as children that food is a source of happiness and celebration at holidays, special occasions, and gatherings in general. I grew up in an Italian family in which food was emphasized in abundance. If you did not have seconds or thirds, there must be a problem. I loved family gatherings with decadent pasta-rich meals and the feeling of stuffing myself with that tasty, comfort-driven food. I also remember feeling *full* of happiness and love at those family meals. Everyone talked loudly; laughter filled the room, and life was simply *good*.

When I began dieting, I became very confused about food. I believed I had to remove the happiness from food and eating because of the restrictive requirements to *fix me* and lose weight. I believed I was supposed to suffer and get used to feeling hungry—really hungry—all the time.

Food and appetite are meant to be savored in a loving, nurturing way to enhance our highest self. This is part of our freakin' human rights! You can achieve it by learning new ways and rewriting your inner script about food. It's time to reclaim your joy and reject the toxicity of dieting.

The Complexity of Hunger

It is so easy to confuse the feeling of *physical* hunger and *emotional* hunger. Common sense says when our stomach growls and our head feels light, our bodies need fuel. That, of course, is physical hunger. Emotional hunger is a desire to fill up on something in our hearts and minds when we are not physically hungry.

Emotional hunger can be misunderstood as a need for comfort foods to provide instant soothing or distraction from an uncomfortable feeling. This misunderstanding is vulnerable to implosion once a dieting belief is set in motion, due to the restricted and deprived mindsets that are required and that do not address emotional connection.

What isn't there enough of in this moment?

What am I trying to avoid?

Since we have discussed appetite, instincts, instant gratification, and happiness, it is clear how easily we can get caught in a vicious cycle of using food to replace or fill up on something missing from our lives. We can use food to hide ourselves from something or someone painful. Whether this comes from an inner rebel or inner protector, food can be a misunderstood, abused tool for self-preservation. And this makes sense, right? Food makes us feel better instantly.

THE CONFUSION FACTORS

The negative body image craze stems from in-your-face media images of retouched, exaggerated photographs and advertisements that can make us want to pack our bags and head for the hills. It takes one seriously self-confident personality not to be impacted by such images. Who doesn't feel the creepy-crawly impact of those judgments and critical thoughts when they see social media posts or ads of those so-called *beautiful* women?

We compare ourselves to those distorted images and swirl in a sea self-loathing, craving chocolate. We also fall prey to believing that the women in the pictures must have *perfect* lives because we see them as having the *perfect* bodies. Adding celebrity diet endorsements to the picture enhances our confusion and desperate sell-out to popular diet programs, so that we can get *their* results and magnificent lives.

In my twelfth year, I was desperately dieting for the perfect body, restricting sugary foods and consuming copious amounts of diet soda and artificial foods. I launched a war with my inner spirit who begged for a reality check and a re-routing back to my authentic self. I was determined to believe the diet culture and shift everything about myself to feel accepted, validated, and loved.

The Deception of Sugar

As mentioned before, sugar is everywhere and has come to symbolize celebration and all things happy. We learn *sugar equals happiness* early in life, and for many of us, this is the budding of a serious problem.

Current data show the typical American consumes six cups of sugar per week, or 152 pounds of sugar per year.[5] This is beyond staggering.

As a kid, I felt I had no control over portions of cookies, cake, and candy. My parents had concerns about my weight, yet sweets showed up everywhere, and somehow the fat kid was supposed to draw up some sort of willpower to have *just a little bit*, or *just moderate her portions*, as if that was so easy. I heard things like, *If you watch what you eat like the other girls do, you can wear all those cute fashions they do.*

It seemed to me like others could have one cookie or eat half their slice of cake or take only a few pieces of Halloween candy, but for me, I just *wanted more.* A lot more. The rebel in me became my Commander in Chief. I remember sneaking more cake when no one was looking, diving into

---

5 New Hampshire Dept. of Health and Human Services. "How Much Sugar Do You Eat?" Health Promotion in Motion. 2014. dhhs.nh.gov/dphs

my brother's Easter basket because I had already eaten all my chocolate, and going into the trash can and pulling out leftover sweets in desperation for *more*.

I grew ashamed and disgusted about my lack of control, and I felt like a slob. I remember my mother being angry with me when I was caught sneaking food and hiding the evidence. Looking back, I had a problem. I was hijacked by habitual consumption and abuse of sugar and processed garbage. My palate and brain chemistry knew no other way but to *scream* for more, like a bratty toddler. But it just made me feel instantly better, every time.

Just a spoonful of sugar makes the medicine go down
The medicine, go dowwwwwn, medicine go down

I may be showing my age by quoting Mary Poppins, but this song subliminally convinced me sugar was a medicinal and loving friend. I often felt it was my only friend.

The Processed Food Revolution

As I was growing up in the 1970s and '80s, sugar and processed foods became mainstream. Fast-food joints became the convenient go-to, feeding the family and making them happy with that satisfying taste.

I remember jumping for joy when it was a McDonald's night or when Mom brought home KFC and all the fixin's. I remember we all gathered around the table, and it was a joyful feast that made everyone happy. A typical lunch was SpaghettiOs or a baloney sandwich on Wonder bread with a hefty side of cheese puffs or chips. Wash it down with red Kool-Aid, which was marketed as so much better than soda. And we *all* ate like this!

Do you remember digging through a box of sugar-loaded crack-cereal to get to the prize? The cereal aisle was two miles long, and TV dinners, Pop-Tarts, microwavable snacks, and more packaged, processed foods exploded onto the market.

Food products and their advertisements were strategically, scientifically designed to trigger our taste buds and brains for addictive behaviors and cravings. This phenomenon hijacked our brains using chemicals, additives, and excessive sugar. Behind the scenes, food marketing and *bliss-point science* went viral, as the goal was to seduce children and parents for profit at the expense of consumer health and sanity.[6] These products are actually anti-foods in the body. They are habit forming, and they draw the tongue away from healthy, natural, whole foods.

The diet revolution came onto the scene with food marketing of fake sugars and processed diet foods. I remember the excitement of diet sodas, sugar-free treats, and diet frozen dinners. What a solution! I consumed processed diet foods with a vengeance, believing exactly what the food marketers

---

6 Moss, Michael. *Salt, Sugar, Fat: How the Food Giants Hooked Us.* Random House, 2014.

wanted me to believe: dieting and consuming diet products would fix me and give me the perfect body.

Truth is, it promoted the exact opposite. I developed a dysfunctional appetite and began some heavily critical self-talk about good food/bad food that I equated to my personal character and integrity. I had no idea what processed food was doing to my brain and my spirit.

What's Wrong With Me?

The battle with dieting, restricting, obsessing, and feeling out of control prompts the frustrating inner questioning of how *normal* people eat to stay at *normal* weight. Add the processed food industry to the mix, and there is now the quandary of what is *normal* food?

Who and what are we supposed to believe?

As a child, I saw so many fast-food restaurants on the highway near my house, I thought if so many of them existed, the food somehow must be good for people to eat.

I grew up in a household where my younger brother was deemed skinny, and I was chubby. My loving, well-meaning parents formed a strategy in which certain foods were for him to beef up and for me to beef down. There was a Hostess outlet in my hometown, and my dad would fill the freezer chock full of Twinkies when they were buy one, get one free.

They were for my brother, and the fruit in the fridge was for me. You can guess how that one went down.

We can laugh about this now, but back then I faced a war zone for me on all levels—physically, mentally, emotionally, and spiritually. The Twinkies took my power with each one—or five—I snarfed down, standing there at the freezer. I was pretty clever at hiding the wrappers. The fruit in the fridge went untouched, of course, even though I did like apples. I usually chose the Twinkie and could never eat just one. Interesting, I do not ever remember bingeing on apples.

You have a powerful story, too, my friend. Reflect on your own history, your food story. Be open to discovering the road map that provides the wisdom and insight for healing your damaged relationship with food, body, and self *the right way*. It begins with openness, willingness, and curiosity about your story.

The upcoming chapters help you in this healing, but for now, it starts with turning inward and reflecting on your magnificent unique food story.

STEP ONE: Discover and Write Your Food Story

This step involves writing about your memories and experiences. Journaling may seem uncomfortable and tedious or may not be your preferred mode of getting clear on your past, but I invite you to give it a try. Do not hold back. This is something private, something just for *you*. This is your chance to signal to your self that you are ready to face and heal your relationship with food *without dieting*.

1. Take a few relaxing moments to sit and reflect. Begin with your earliest childhood memories of eating and, perhaps, where you were and what foods were present. Pay particular attention to your first memories of eating that made you feel happy or loved.

2. Use a journal or open a document on your computer and begin writing or typing freely. This is for you, so no worries about spelling or proper punctuation. Simply allow your thoughts to flow onto the document. For example, you may remember a birthday party, family dinner, or holiday celebration. Write your feelings and what you remember eating.

3. Record your memories in your stages of growth and how you remember yourself as an eater. Record memories that relate to how you felt in your body, how you understood your hunger, and whether you remember experiencing confusion or problems that related to food or your patterns with eating.

4. Give yourself plenty of quiet, open space and time to do this. You may be surprised at the emotions that come up as well as the length of your food story.

5. Where you choose to stop is up to you; however, it is a good idea to write as much as you can remember.

> You could even reflect on your food habits all the way up to your decision to read this book.

This was the first step in my own therapy of reclaiming my life as it relates to food, body, and self. I love occasionally going back and reading my story. I laugh and cry and grow stronger each time.

I am excited for you to begin to process *your* story.

CHAPTER TWO

The Shift

ABANDONING THE SPIRIT; AWAKENING THE BEAST

We are born knowing instinctively when we have had enough to eat.

We express emotions and process responses from others. Depending on our early environment, many of us may have discovered that expressing feelings and emotions can be unsafe and should be held in, so as not to make other people uncomfortable or to avoid getting a hurtful reaction.

We may begin deeply integrating instructions from our caregivers, such as:

- Follow the rules.
- Be a good girl.
- Be quiet.
- Do what is expected, and you'll be praised.

This is when many of us leave our bodies behind and get into our heads, where we develop interior voices. Those of us who, as small children, developed an exaggerated sense of food being connected to love and safety tend to put this emotional tool into our little backpack and shoulder it as we evolve into the next stage of life.

Puberty is like the Wild Mouse ride at a carnival, where we are spinning around fast with no clear path. We are, in many ways, all alone in our heads. Things go well for some and not for others. Some of us are taught to believe that feelings and emotions are signs of weakness, have little to no meaning, and should be ignored. *No one likes a crybaby. Only the tough survive.*

I had a fighter inside of me, so I bought in to this theory early on. Beliefs in this stage are built hard and fast from a physiological, biological, and emotional perspective. We find ourselves growing at a pace faster than we can control. For some, this is an exciting time of what seems like unending social acceptance and elevation from family and peers. But for many others, especially the identified *chubby girl*, this only strengthens the internal war with self, in which food becomes the bandage for wounds and the secret weapon for protection. We seek instant comfort from food, which seems like the only truly reliable source of nurturance, safety, and love. But its comfort is only temporary, just a Band-Aid.

The Imprinted Beliefs

Who invented the ridiculous notion that children should be seen and not heard?

I believe this can be a stinger to the hearts of children who hear these words at an early age. Of course, children need to be taught appropriate manners and polite graces; however, children who were told that they should not be heard can often internalize this as *I am not worthy, important, or acceptable*—that they do not matter.

If children sense that they are not acceptable, not enough, or that they are, on some level, *unsafe*, food can quickly become the friend for instant relief of heavy emotions. Food often feels as though it is the only reliable, consistent source of comfort, love, and acceptance. The dysfunctional relationship with food creates the conditions for a self-sabotaging battle of food, body, and self.

When I was a child, no one seemed to understand my appetite—least of all, me. As my reliance on sugar intensified, so did my feelings of being unworthy, unaccepted, and not enough. No one wants to see, hear, or validate a chubby girl who obviously has no self-control or willpower. She is labeled as *lazy, gross,* and *someone who just eats too much*. My main source of validation came from comparing myself to other girls who were bigger than me. That somehow gave me confirmation that I wasn't that far off the rails.

The Judge and the Label

Ultimately, we all want love in our lives, don't we?

Everyone wants to be loved, no matter what—to feel deeply as though someone has our back. We don't want to feel judged by our appearance, mistakes, talents or lack thereof, accomplishments, status, weight, shape, size, quality of clothing, house we live in, car we drive, on so on. We crave outside approval and affirmation that we are going to be okay in this world and that we are worthy, loveable, and enough *as is*.

When children are supported by unconditional love, they have a foundation on which they can develop self-trust and belief in themselves. This is an invincible shield for protecting one's spirit. As a chubby girl, I felt loved, but frequent expressions of well-meaning concerns from my loving parents prompted the feeling of being labeled, as if I wore a banner on my forehead that read:

TRACY EATS TOO MUCH.

This fortified the belief I was building that my chubby appearance somehow advertised a massive fault in my character. My childhood reliance on junk food as my go-to for relieving discomfort and pain grew through high school.

The Former Free Spirit

Was there a time in your life when you felt free to just be yourself, when you were comfortable being the real you, and life felt open and unencumbered by negative thoughts of self?

Maybe when you felt your appetite was natural and you were not obsessing about food or your body, or perhaps before giving a rat's ass about *fitting in* or what size you wore?

What did you love doing as a child when you didn't have a care in the world?

I remember my childhood days before I fell prey to body image and dieting. I was a free-spirited little girl who loved to celebrate the simple joys in life: friends, disco music, roller-skating, food, and laughing without barriers.

In fourth grade, I was the class clown, the creative, loud-mouth persona who would do just about anything to make others laugh, especially during boring school. I frequently was sent to the principal's office because of my disruptive antics and uncontrollable laughter in the classroom. Even with those consequences, cracking up with my peers was always worth it. This was me being my rule-breaking, unapologetic self who loved initiating joy, laughter, and happiness with others.

I was confident and I liked myself.

I was too chubby to wear *normal* clothes, so I was relegated to shopping in the "Pretty Plus" section of JC Penney's. My polyester pants clung tightly, yet comfortably, to my robust rear end. The fabric of the inner thighs was well worn and pilled from the friction of my thighs rubbing together. I was a bit too chubby for those designer blue jeans that were becoming all the rage, but I made the most of those stretchy pants—especially when worn with a loose, flowy, matching top with an embroidered roller skate on it or an iron-on of Donny and Marie.

I always had the feeling that my thin mother was embarrassed by my unpopular plus-sized fashion needs for my plump body, but my free-spirited inner rebel sported a WTF mentality and donned those elastic-waisted polyester pants with pride. I even discovered a trick with those stretchy pants that I used to my advantage many times.

They were great for getting a running start, slamming down on my knees on the linoleum floor and sliding all the way down the hall after lunch in front of all my classmates who were quietly following the rules and lining up along the wall waiting for the teacher. They all laughed hysterically at me.

I loved making others laugh, which brought sunshine into the world—that was my gift. What better medicine is there than laughter that makes your belly hurt in a good way? I felt immensely fulfilled when I made other people smile and feel happy. This was truly me, alive in my spirit. Life was good.

That was what I like to describe as *the calm before the storm.*

I left my confident badass fourth grader behind in 1980. I became prey to what would become decades of body image obsession and dieting to become someone else, to fix and change who I was. Girls who had perfect hair and the perfect ass to fill out the designer painted-on jeans were admired, respected, and loved by everyone, especially boys. My polyester pants were now a huge embarrassment, and I lost my confidence in my ability to make others laugh. This was *no longer enough*, and I was not enough.

I believed that to fit in, I had to be different than I was. I had to be thin, talented, and good at sports, which I wasn't. Otherwise, I believed I was failing. And a free-spirit rebel of a kid *does not fail.* She fights relentlessly.

I was hell-bent on fitting in, so I formed a new strategy of stuffing my ass into those designer jeans and cuffing the extra fabric at the bottom of those bastards to account for the extra room needed for my beefiness. I stuffed my bra, put on excessive makeup, and prayed for my hair to behave each morning so I could get that perfect feathery look.

THE SELL-OUT TO IDEOLOGY

Something happens, particularly to girls, in that dreaded preteen phase. It is like a tidal wave of change, biologically and psychologically. It can feel like our own *Jurassic Park*, where we wander in uncharted territory, hoping to fit in and not encounter scary monsters who threaten our very survival.

We take notice of society's standards of success and admiration. We then give birth to an inner critical voice and the constant chatter of assessment of self for such standards. *Fasten your seat belt, Chubby Girl; you're in for a bumpy ride.* I was.

The Priceless Trade-In

My Pretty-Plus badass self took a big hit one Saturday morning in sixth grade. I was in my Catechism class, and for some reason, the heavy classroom door became jammed shut and would not budge when it was time to leave. We were all stuck in that classroom and were forced to wait until the fire department got there to rescue us.

One by one, we were instructed to line up by the door and step on a chair to be lifted and pulled out of the glass section of the heavy wooden door that the firemen had smashed through. When it was my turn, I stepped onto the chair, and one of the fire men reached to pull me out. He announced, "Okay, here comes a *big one!*" I felt a dagger in my heart that scarred me in ways I would not discover until decades later.

I believed dieting was my ticket to attaining the slim shape I coveted. I drank diet sodas and choked down skim milk and Crystal Light drinks. I ate plain crackers, carrots, tuna, hard-boiled eggs, and frozen diet entrees. I restricted all junk foods and tried to force myself to get used to being hungry all the time. I was pushing for willpower, which was supposed to be the golden tool.

This was a true recipe for disaster. Diets rob our souls and make us crazy. They strip us of the inner gifts we have been given to share in this life by demanding our attention for rules and restrictions.

My parents were loving and well-meaning and did the best they could, based on what they truly believed. As a parent with two grown children, I understand parenting is a tough job. Their attempts to motivate me to watch what I ate, on occasion, using destructive, critical language only polarized my inner rebel and left scars. I ended up bolting to food for relief and escape.

I felt as though I needed to punish myself for my lack of self-control. These were the comfort and soothing tools in the emotional backpack I carried around in my subconscious throughout childhood. *Feel bad—eat food, mainly sugar—feel better*. I was developing a habitual, toxic reliance on sugar that trained my brain for decades of suffering to come. Part of me was like a toxic beast, and its language played on repeat in my mind. I really believed I had a shameful, embarrassing problem that no one else had with food. I believed there was innately something wrong with me and these toxic beliefs about my personal character began draining my self-image and self-respect.

The Desperate Search for Enoughness

I gave up on myself in the chase after a skinny and beautiful, fixed body. The perfect body seemed impossible to achieve. I felt helpless to fit in and to feel like I was somehow *enough* to have friends and some version of success, or validation, in the world.

Society pushed images that *thin was in*. I also knew deep down inside that this wasn't *me*. I wasn't thin. Did I really even *care* to be? My former fourth-grade, badass, Pretty-Plus-self whom I once liked was not enough and was certainly not in. I felt ashamed of her, so I ignored her. The truth was, I was secretly ignoring my spirit.

The pop media of the 1980s told us to *slim down*. I thought it was my ticket to fitting in. Restricting myself from tasty food and ignoring my gnawing hunger created a feeling of suffering and confusion that was overwhelming. Sugar and my inner rebel became next-level besties because, when the pressure of life and dieting became suffocating, we would party on in private with instant WTF relief from *all of it*.

I built an invisible tidal wave of shame and disgust inside my emotional mind and heart that hurt all the time. The fighter in me felt ultimately defeated with each binge that left me with only a few pairs of pants I could fit into.

I was told I had *such a pretty face*, and I should be able to wear the fashions that the other girls wore. This landed on me as more failure, more confirmation that, somehow, I was not enough. The fighter in me took over. I was a survivor. The protector of my heart took over and chose a scary path from then on: more dieting.

Burgeoning Insanity

We dieters develop a voice inside that trumps our common sense. We learn to label our entire freakin' character as *good or bad, success or failure*, all based on our perception of whether we are following through on our diet—and, of course, what we see on the scale.

The game of dieting sucks the life out of us at a level we do not comprehend. The amount of mental energy that is required in this chase is mind-boggling and robs us of precious time spent on other valuable, fulfilling life ventures and our God-given purpose.

Think of the emotions and feelings you have when you vow to *start over on Monday* in your chosen diet. You trick yourself into believing the postponed rescue mission of starting over on your diet.

How many times have you done this?

You eat something *off plan* or *ate too many points*, feel like you failed, go off the rails and binge, then criticize yourself with toxic lingo in your head. This dissonance only exacerbates and validates the space for binge eating, time and time again. And the insanity of this is that we believe there is no other way. Just start over, and . . . do the same thing. Try harder, with more willpower, or maybe spend hundreds of dollars on the new popular plan with supplements or fake food. *Anything* for hope. *Anything* but the truth and common sense.

This is what I think all the letters of the word *diet* stand for:

> **D**eprivation
>
> **I**nsanity
>
> **E**quals
>
> **T**rouble

Truth be told, my former free spirit knew dieting was insane and that there had to be a better way. Since I hid my dysfunction with food, I simply surged forward, trying the same dieting tactics over and over.

The real me inside kicked, screamed, and rebelled with food binges. I would eat so much that I did not have an appetite for dinner and would need to lie down for hours. Bingeing on sugar and carbs was my only escape most days, in the afternoons when my inner rebel took over. Although I turned to them to relieve my pain, these binges were controlling me, and I felt powerless. Layers of character flaw, shame, and demoralization grew.

To protect this uncontrollable shame, I decided I should play it safe and small and protect myself from anything that would cause me to feel the sting of failure and rejection. The only true source of comfort was my secret life with sugar and junk food and the temporarily insane yet reliable relief it provided me.

I was trapped in an endless hell of fighting with diets that did not serve me and tactics that were not sustainable.

My college years and early adulthood were consumed with more inner fighting and dieting. My arsenal included fat-free foods like plain bagels, hard pretzels, and sugary cereals in bulk, excessive diet soda, artificial sweeteners, and l-i-t-e junk foods. I purchased TV-advertised programs like "Stop the Insanity" and ate fat-free because, as it was advertised, "the fat makes you fat." Add excessive aerobic exercise to my strategy of restriction and control, and my life of cyclical bingeing and exercising continued.

My binge eating persisted for the next two decades, as I fought myself with restrictive food plans. My desperation even sparked a bizarre jealousy for girls I knew who were battling anorexia or bulimia. I believed they had more *hard willpower* than me. I just pigged out all the time.

There appeared to be no recognition or identified help for people like me who binged but did not purge or starve themselves. This sent the message that we must just be weak or have no willpower. *Just go find the next diet and try harder.* Good luck with that. This is an example of how dieting makes us crazy and robs our common sense and sanity. It strips us of the inner gifts we have been given to share with the world.

It distracts us with rules that claim to give us weight loss, the perfect body, and the perfect life. This is not true, and it never ends well.

The media and diet culture lure us into the perception that having a perfect, thin body is the secret to a happy, abundant, perfect life.

Do we really think we were put on this Earth to diet and regain weight over and over?

Do we not have a greater purpose to fulfill?

LOSS OF SELF-TRUST

I remembered somewhere in my intrinsic heart that I was a fighter. I could change and control my situation if I really wanted to. I remember the words: *You can have anything you want in life if you want it bad enough.*

Dieting promised a dream. It was the ultimate solution for weight loss, according to all the magazines and TV. Give up and restrict all my favorite foods and suffer until I see a number on the scale. That was the only solution. I believed if I could just learn to live with the discomfort of being hungry most of the time and ignore my appetite, I would get thin and I would magically be loved, accepted, and successful; then my life would transform into my dream come true. Meanwhile, my spirit screamed for truths that I ignored.

The natural, innate appetite for nourishment we were born with becomes a thing of the past. Dieting teaches us to take on toxic thoughts about food, our bodies, and ultimately our measure of worth. We buy into the lie that our value is assessed by our appearance. Social media suffocates us with images of perceived perfection.

I felt like one giant loser every time I attempted a new diet and quickly failed with a rebellious binge. Each time this happened, I developed toxic beliefs about myself which equated to the notion that I could no longer trust myself—in essence, I became detached from my former free spirit who used to be confident and trusted in my Self.

Here is where we disconnect from ourselves. We lose common sense, self-trust, natural appetite regulation, and self-awareness in the game of dieting. I forgot what it had felt like to eat when my body was truly hungry and to stop when I naturally felt satisfied, not stuffed.

Chutes & Ladders

The battleground of dieting reminded me of a giant game of Chutes & Ladders. Remember the board game from Milton Bradley?

When we diet, we flick the spinner and hope to land on ladder spots so we can quickly climb all the way to the top by means restricting food and following rules. At some point, we grow tired and bored of playing. We flick the spinner again and land on a chute, eating a treat that's off-plan. *BAM!* We perceive failure and sliiiiiide down that chute all the way to the bottom. Defeated, we start all over again in an insane repetitive diet. This is all we know. This time we will try harder. Flick the damn spinner again and hope for a better outcome.

Dieting promotes an out-of-body experience in which we surrender our instincts, common sense, and intuition about food. Instead, we follow a chosen set of rules that sell us on weight-loss results, a better body, and, ultimately, a better life.

When our intuition begs for attention by fighting the rules, we abandon the diet, rebel and binge, and convince ourselves that next time, with more willpower, we'll do better. But until then, party on! We surrender our birthright sanity with this insidious belief that dieting is our solution and our intuition deep within is wrong.

Points to Ponder

When did your dieting game begin in your food story?

Assuming you have completed your *Step One: Discover and Write Your Food Story*, take a moment to remember at what point did you begin a popular commercial diet? Perhaps you restricted food on your own terms. Maybe you remember simply beginning to control or fight yourself over your favorite foods in general and felt a sense of powerlessness.

Reflect on how it felt for you emotionally when you began dieting, perhaps what form of diet or restriction it was, how this felt for you at the time, and what happened as a result. What takeaways did you remember having about those experiences?

Write them as a side note page in your food story. Remember, this is private, for only you to see, and is a very powerful activity to begin building your self-awareness within your food story history for the exciting healing steps ahead.

Do you remember how old you were when you began dieting or following restrictive food programs?

I followed popular themes like:

- Fat-free
- Low carb
- Low-calorie
- Ketogenic
- Sugar-free
- High protein
- Cleanses
- Detoxes
- Weight Watchers (WW)

Plus, I followed my own plan of restriction.

Write down all you can remember about the details: how you felt, the results you experienced, and what happened for you afterward.

Did you sustain results? If so, for how long?

Did you try one of the above programs, give up, then try that same one or a different program?

These examples of questions to consider are identifications for yourself that set the stage for the healing steps ahead.

All these dieting strategies had a start date and a future date upon which I set a goal for my final weigh-in and goal weight achievement—an event that rarely happened, by the way. I often hit my chart-imposed goal weight, but I never kept my results very long because I could not sustain the warpath diet tactics it took to get me there.

My body suffered in my battle of chronic dieting, bingeing on sugar, and eating processed foods. I experienced hormone irregularity, brain chemistry irregularities, stress, radical mood swings, weight fluctuations, and serious macronutrient imbalance.

I had no concept of how to nourish my body. This led to more intense cravings, feelings of habituated reliance and addictions to sugar and carbs, poor sleep cycles, out-of-control bingeing, recovering, dieting, and starting over. No one knew as my body was punished, my spirit was dying. The dieting game was killing me from the inside out.

I needed help with this inner war I was fighting with food and myself, but I was too embarrassed and ashamed at that time. I simply labeled myself as someone who was weak and had no willpower with food.

If you identify with these challenges in your own food story, never fear! As explained before, Step One is identifying, writing, reflecting, and processing your food story from your past up through the present. Assuming you have completed this step, it is now time to get acquainted with yourself again, or perhaps for the first time, and begin designing your healing new food story that elevates your life on your chosen terms.

THE BREAKTHROUGH

Americans alone spend $33 billion each year on weight-loss products, fueling that ever-booming, profit-driven diet industry.[7] Sadly, we also spend years of our intrinsically more costly and precious mental and emotional energy. We fight ourselves to achieve some version of a better body, which we are lured into believing will magically produce a better life.

Consider how many years you may have been focusing on dieting. When I reflect on my own life, I feel tremendously sad at the thought of what I spent energetically on this ridiculous chase. I remember having the thought: *When I get control over my eating habits, I can take on (this or that) goal, but first, I need to tweak my eating plan and lose x number of pounds.*

---

7 bmc.org/nutrition-and-weight-management/weight-management

And then I will be happy with myself and my life, and somehow it will all just get better.

The chase prompts the toxic belief that our happiness with ourselves and our lives should be delegated to the future until we lose weight and win the gold medal. I have hit my goal weight a few times, but it has been from relentless combat with myself over food, exercise, and the scale. I went so far as to use laxatives on my weigh-in day. That is no way to live, mind you.

And guess what? I was no happier.

In fact, at times, I felt like a panicked, caged rebel who won something inauthentic that I knew I could not hold on to. I was one cookie away from a binge from hell.

The act of dieting is one giant stressor. We begin a diet with a euphoric honeymoon feeling of excitement and the hope of our weight-loss dream coming true. The truth is that dieting is a stress response that *fuels the desire* to use food to cope and downshift our metabolic furnace to protect our reserves. We become disconnected with ourselves as a result.

My friends, if this resonates with you, please know there is a pathway out of postponing your happiness. The remaining chapters in this book address healing this toxic, limiting belief pattern. You can learn to break free of the patterns that keep you stuck, holding on to thoughts about yourself that are overly comfortable and that reference the past, not the future.

Decide now to allow yourself happiness *just as you are right now*. If you feel like swearing at me, I get it.

You may be asking: *How can you tell me to feel happy when I feel fat, bloated, depressed, disconnected, and horrible in my body?*

I get it. This was me. This is a great example of how the game of dieting robs us of more spiritual gifts than we can consciously understand. Fortunately, there is a simple way we can accept ourselves in the present and see past the incessant inner pressure, noise, and self-imposed contingencies of fixing ourselves for future outcomes before we allow ourselves to feel worthy of happiness.

Stop.

Be present and think of three things in any given moment that you are truly grateful for. I am not kidding. The power of gratitude is a real thing. By taking moments in your day to see what is good in your life right now, you begin to train your mind to seek the good and allow yourself to be happy in your body right now, not postpone your happiness until you *get the weight off*.

Friends, you can always find three things you are grateful for in any given moment. Even on the bad days. In fact, most of the time, when I practice this, my three things are extremely simple and come to mind quickly. Right now, I am grateful for the cool breeze coming through my window as I type, the hot coffee sitting on my desk making me feel alert, and my husband, who gave me a genuine hug when I left home today.

Taking time to pause in any moment in your day to recognize, from your heart, three simple things you are grateful for gives you an opportunity to feel instant peace and happiness, with no future contingencies. Intentionally practicing this each day helps us to shift into a more positive mindset about ourselves and our circumstances and sets the tone for inner healing with optimism and enlightenment about ourselves and our lives.

Please be open to the healing thought that our way out of the diet prison begins in a place of loving compassion, not judgment, criticism, or fighting with yourself. Those things never serve us.

A secret to finding peace with food, body, and self begins with our hearts. We must be willing to loosen our grip on dieting and to look inward with a sense of calm and curiosity. Give yourself permission to simply feel happy in the now, with no future contingencies.

At this point, take deep breath, exhale, and relax into this super fun next step where you begin to uncover the real *you* on the inside.

Your Diva Discovered

What do I mean by *Diva?*

A Diva can be expressed in a variety of ways. For purposes of this book, however, a Diva shall refer to the no-nonsense woman who takes full responsibility for owning her place and purpose in the world and knows what she is all about. She accepts and trusts herself, is confident, and is not afraid of hard work. She emulates inner peace and has no need for external validation from the world.

A *Diet-Free Diva* is a woman who knows what she intrinsically needs for holistic nourishment of her mind, body, and spirit. She designs her life accordingly.

Chasing a false sense of worth and identity, as we do when we diet, is exhausting. We lose track of the things that drive us to be alive. We forget what makes us happy and joyful, and we become disconnected from our spirit, which is the beacon of clarity for our life's purpose. Our way out of this personal dieting war is to take back our ability to live *embodied*—to turn inward and discover motivational markers.

What truly drives us from within with passion, tenacity, and authenticity to find our *Diva?*

When she is at her best, pursuing her life mission, your Diva is serving others at a high level. She rocks out her best self, and that makes the world a better place. She loves, respects, and trusts herself and, therefore, others.

We all have an inner Diva who is the best version of ourselves in mind, body, and spirit.

What is the reason or purpose of living your Best Diva Life?

Try the following steps to discover what makes you tick. This is also a major part of your *why* for living your Best Diva Life and breaking free from the destructive, debilitating chase of dieting.

STEP TWO: Identify Your Top Three Values and Write Your Personal Powerful Why (PPW)

Part A: You can heal your soul from the battering it has taken while dieting.

Turn inward, settle yourself, and ask these questions:

- *What do I value most?*
- *What are the most important aspects of living my life to the fullest?*
- *What makes me unique?*

Another way to discover your values is to ask simply: *What is important to me?*

Check out this chart below and circle your intrinsic top values.

This forms the framework to design your healing pathway *out* of dieting and *into* nourishing yourself from the inside out, claiming your authentic life on your own badass terms.

This is not easy because we often hear the word *should* creeping into our heads. What we *should* think or do is usually based on what we think society and others want from us. Instead, listen for your own wisdom and ponder deeply who you truly are and *what you want.*

It may feel overwhelming or daunting to do this. If this is true for you, try narrowing your responses to just three values. When I dove into my heart and really thought about this, I discovered that I love:

1. Feeling healthy and energetic (health)
2. Being independently creative (freedom)
3. Doing fulfilling work that contributes to the greater good (fulfillment)

Those are my Top Three Values that I now use to design my life on *my* terms.

List of Values

Abundance	Connection	Family	Independence	Parenting	Self-respect
Accountability	Contentment	Financial security	Integrity	Passion	Service
Achievement	Contribution	Flexibility	Intelligence	Patience	Spirituality
Adventure	Courage	Forgiveness	Intuition	Peace	Success
Ambition	Creativity	Freedom	Job security	Perseverance	Teamwork
Authenticity	Curiosity	Friendship	Joy	Personal development	Thriftiness
Balance	Dedication	Fulfillment	Justice	Playfulness	Thoughtfulness
Beauty	Dependability	Fun	Kindness	Power	Tradition
Belonging	Dignity	Generosity	Knowledge	Proactivity	Travel
Calmness	Diversity	Gratitude	Leadership	Professionalism	Trust
Career	Education	Growth	Learning	Recognition	Truth
Challenge	Efficiency	Happiness	Legacy	Resilience	Understanding
Change	Empathy	Health	Love	Respect	Uniqueness
Collaboration	Enthusiasm	Home	Loyalty	Responsibility	Vision
Commitment	Environment	Honesty	Mindfulness	Risk-taking	Wealth

Com-munity	Equality	Humility	Motiva-tion	Safety	List your own:
Com-passion	Ethics	Humor	Opti-mism	Security	______
Compe-tence	Excel-lence	Impact	Order	Self-dis-cipline	______
Confi-dence	Faith	Inclu-sion	Nature	Self-ex-pression	______

Part B: Once you've identified your priorities, you can focus on your motivational target and begin to understand what drives you from within and what is most important to you, deep down inside. Knowing yourself innately and what drives you forms the initial framework the next step, asking yourself some important questions to build motivation and clarity for moving forward and making powerful habit changes. You'll have a target to aim for. This bull's eye is your very own *Personal Powerful Why*, or PPW.

Let's be clear on this. You may have heard of finding your *why* in other books or interviews with success coaches.

Why is everyone talking about this?

Because it is *that important*. This was a revelation to me. I had gotten this so wrong—I had failed to connect to myself and what really mattered to me, not what the world or anyone else said or implied should matter to me. Once you know your top values, you can envision yourself living your Best Diva Life.

Dream here, friends, because this is totally within your reach, if you commit to finding the real bull's eye.

You can:

- Break free from dieting.
- Lose your unwanted pounds.
- Improve your energy.
- Feel vibrant.
- Harness your Best Diva Life in a sustainable way.

I needed to honor my PPW so I could find the courage to write this book for you. That required me to tackle a fear and further positive change for other women who share my battles with dieting.

So, now it's your turn.

Part C: Next, envision your Best Diva Self, living these values in your daily life. Consider these questions carefully, and write your answers.

What do you need to shift?

What does that look like and feel like to you?

Why do you want to learn ways to break free from dieting for good?

***So you can*________________.**

***Then you'd have*________________.**

***To do (what and why)?*____________________.**

When I got clear on my Top Three Values (health, independence, fulfillment), I understood my decisions and actions needed to align with what I valued most, in order to live a vibrant, Best Diva Life.

I also knew that my battle with dieting had no place in my life and that I needed to face what was asking for attention to move in the direction of honoring myself and creating the abundant life I was meant to live on my unique terms. I had to get clear on *why* I wanted to stop the war with food and diets and figure out how to eat to nourish my entire life, not just to lose weight.

I envisioned myself as my Best Diva Self, living out my values in abundance. I then asked myself the above questions:

What do I need to shift?

My controlling battle with food and dieting.

What does that look and feel like to me?

It feels free and liberating to find trust with food and, more importantly, with myself.

Why do I want to learn ways to break free from dieting for good?

Because I realize how much precious energy I have been spending on the diet fight. This energy is taking away from things I want to pursue in my life, like writing and speaking with confidence. I realize how trapped I have become inside myself. I wanted out.

So I can: trust myself with food and have the confidence, clarity, and mental space to then pursue meaningful endeavors that align with my purpose, my values, and my Best Diva Self; for example, writing this book.

Then I'd have: the benefit of all my favorite clothes in my closet fitting me consistently and not holding on to the *someday* too-tight clothes.

To do (what and why)? To live my life on my confident, trusted terms because this is true freedom.

Keep your answers brief and be impeccably honest with yourself. You will need to remember your PPW in weak moments, and you will have plenty of those on your journey. We all do. Remembering why you are saying no to some things and yes to other things, and to align with your values, your PPW must be front and center in your mind—or the temptations will become overpowering.

Well done! So far you have completed some powerful self-discovery work that I hope has given you an opportunity to reflect on where you have come in your life (your food story) and where you are right now. You have also identified what is most important to you (values) and why you want to break free from dieting (PPW) to live your Best Diva Life, which you have envisioned.

You are now ready to move forward with the next exciting steps in healing.

Onward!

CHAPTER THREE

The Fork In The Road

RECLAIMING YOUR POWER

When we take the time to read our food story, reflect on our experiences with dieting, and see the emotional challenges that were created with these roots, we give ourselves space for curiosity and compassion. We believed what we knew at the time. We tried hard. We did not fail. Diets failed us.

We learned valuable lessons about ourselves—lessons that we embrace with gratitude for bringing us to the right here and now. We have the power to decide how to live our lives on our terms, especially related to our choices with food. It is time to create our future food story by reclaiming our power that we gave to diet culture and trusting we have our answers to a peaceful relationship with food inside us right now. It is time to find answers and put them into action on our terms.

Princess Becomes Queen

Dieting keeps us stuck in a fantasy-like *Princess* mode, according to Marc David of the Institute for the Psychology of Eating. Princess mode relies on external validation for approval from the world. In this world, we chase body image, our goal weight, and external validation based on appearance. We desperately want to know that the world considers us to be *enough*. Social media further casts visions of what is deemed acceptable, beautiful, and worthy, according to society.

Understanding how diet culture can contribute to emotional wounds that take root in our relationship with ourselves, we can then see this challenge for what it is—false toxic programming. It is time to elevate out of Princess mode and into our Queen mode. Your Queen-self emulates your purposeful, badass, Best Diva Self in mind, body, and spirit on a holistic level. You've already taken the initial steps toward this major shift by defining your highest values and tapping in to your inner authentic spirit for healing.

In a state of true overall mature wellness, you have reclaimed your power on your terms. You've gathered tools that build your self-trust and self-respect, perhaps the very ones you previously traded in during your dieting. You develop a no-bullshit, elevated attitude about yourself and how you rock your world on your terms. There is no doubt; you know it on a deep, unshakable level. There is no need for external validation because you have your own.

Deep down, you know your truth. You are entitled to discover and honor these truths because you are a unique individual and a magnificent human being, alive on planet Earth with a divine purpose to be discovered and cultivated for the greater good.

Our work together now is to release and heal the toxicity of limiting beliefs that are often rooted in painful early life experiences. There is a calling from within that knows what is best for you in your relationship with food, body, and self. It is time to make space for this healing and to take back your freedom to be your authentic self. We have inside us all the tools we need to establish effective freedom. We must go inward and claim them like never before.

You have identified your Top Three Values; the next step is to practice honoring them. When you honor your values, you may find yourself developing new beliefs. You are, in effect, teaching yourself that you are more trustworthy and more valuable. You can initiate designing your life to support your inner spirit in a wholesome, nurturing manner. All of a sudden, you just might find joy in living your life fully rather than only in food.

Food used to be my only source of joy. Then I connected with who I am by identifying what I value most. I learned to think differently to heal and find peace in my life without abusing food. I discovered a fresh perspective that paved the road for healing my old relationship with food that had held me captive. The shift occurred for me only when I opened my mind, softened my heart, and allowed God, my inner wisdom, to take the driver's seat. I became curious rather than defensive and limited in my thinking. I gave myself permission to let go of white knuckling my way through my inner world.

Vitamin L: *Love*

Deciding to break free from dieting is a courageous decision that can be scary. We find ourselves entering new territory and can feel helpless when we stop following the rules and restrictions of a diet.

To step into your Queen, embrace the concepts that you are enough, you are valid, and you are worthy as a woman right now, as is—period—with no conditions or contingencies. When we can do this, we become open to loving ourselves for who we are. This is an essential vitamin for healing from within, vitamin L, *love.*

Healing comes from connecting with your heart, loving yourself right now—just as you are—and committing to honor your values and decisions to live your life on your terms, rooted in your PPW. Your unique values, when honored, will help you achieve freedom and confidence. You are living an authentic life. In this way, we graduate from little girl and Princess to mature woman and Queen.

How can you reclaim your power?

Be in your body; love your body *right now*. Believe in the power you possess to honor your life according to your values. Allow your heart to heal from the inside. You will mature into who you are meant to be.

Believe that you are not broken; you are not a problem to be fixed. You are a beautiful soul who is worthy of peace, love, and healing.

Embrace vitamin L. Discover how loving ourselves provides open space for allowing your inner wisdom and answers become clear to you. The pathway to heal a damaged relationship with food must begin with cultivating self-love in place of the inner war that is associated with dieting.

Beautiful Permission

I would like to share an example of how choosing to embrace Vitamin L and unconditionally loving our body in the now can result in a surprising boost of happy sunshine. Sometimes we simply need to give ourselves beautiful permission to love ourselves in our bodies right now.

When I worked as a personal trainer, I had an orientation meeting with a delightful woman I'll call "Joyce," who was considering working with me. Joyce was down on herself. She shared her heartfelt struggles and shame for having gained so much weight. I felt her pain, and I understood this sense of deflation and withdrawal.

Joyce was struggling with her relationship with food and her body. She was hoping I could design an exercise program for her so she could change her body and get happy. I paused in thought, and with compassion, I encouraged her to think more gently about her life and herself. I gave her an assignment. I told her that, before we began her exercise programming, I wanted her to go shopping for some new exercise clothes that fit her and made her feel comfortable and attractive in her body *right now*. Then we would begin her exercise together.

Her face lit up like a Christmas tree because I was asking her first to love and accept herself as is, somehow giving her permission to feel happy right now. This would make the next step in healing her physical body more open and nurturing. She signed up for personal training with me, and we began a heartfelt training relationship together that was founded in loving connection more than in the act of exercising.

For today, we will start small together by giving ourselves beautiful permission for loving actions toward ourselves. We'll seek happiness *as we are, right now,* without criticisms, comparisons, or judgments. Gratitude for our amazing hearts and what is good, *right now,* about us and our lives is fuel that powers us along the healing road ahead.

TO STAY OR TO LAUNCH

It is now time for an honest reality check. If you make no changes, you are saying yes to your habits, to your comforts, and to your existing level of health and well-being. I have no judgment here; I'm simply asking how you feel in your current relationship with food, body, and self.

If you are ready to say yes to trying new self-nurturing ideas that will give you the opportunity to explore who you are when you are not fighting with food, then make the commitment to yourself that you will give your honest, best efforts with the upcoming steps.

Face yourself, right now, where you are, with your current habits and relationship with food, body, and self. I am guessing that this book attracted you because you are seeking some no-nonsense, diet-free strategies to find sustainable peace with food and to improve your health. You are ready to say no to lies and the façade of dieting culture and yes to the truth and the right way to eat, to live, and to thrive as your *best*.

The Comfort Zone

Dieting can be an addictive force or comfort zone in which we associate the euphoric restart of a diet and way of life. You may have had success with a certain diet in the past. We can develop a habituated return to the same diet because we believe it worked for us and made us feel temporarily great.

We blame ourselves for the failure of this plan and vow that next time we'll try harder.

Because we were able to get results before, for however a brief time, we think this particular plan works—and it's the only plan that will work for us. Well, *enough of that!* I have battled my way to goal weight on many occasions and kept my so-called results for, maybe, one week until I rebelled and began bingeing again. I'm not sure we can call that actually *working*, however. I believed at the time that it did work, but it was killing me from the inside out.

To move away from the diet mentality, one must be open and curious to a new approach. It may feel odd to reject diet plan rules, regulations, scales, and lies, particularly if you have a long history of having relied on this way of thinking. But you are learning a new way of being and moving through the world. That requires some patience with yourself. Try to suspend judgment long enough to develop new behaviors and beliefs.

The active approach is a no-deadline system of small, customized, doable steps that have a one-day-at-a-time focus with a ton of mindful self-connection.

- Are you willing to consider that you can find joy, comfort, and happiness in sources other than your favorite go-to foods?

- Are you willing to consider tools to help with cravings and emotional connection that will give you the power to stop bolting to food to escape, numb, or cope?
- Are you willing to be uncomfortable in the onset of learning a new skill of nourishing yourself holistically?
- Are you willing to give yourself a chance rather than believe in yet another diet attempt that will fail you?

It can be scary to give up the habit of using food as an emotional escape, like breaking up with a best friend. This can leave a binge eater with a subconscious void. We fill the void by holding on to certain diet plans or foods because we believe we need them. We compensate in other ways—maybe keeping those candy-bar-diet-liar-protein-bars or shakes because they *satisfy a sweet tooth.* We make up for this by skipping meals, over-exercising, or other methods of control to keep our comfy friends around.

This only keeps us stuck in a dysfunctional reliance on food for comfort and will not ultimately serve our greater good in healing what is truly calling us. Courage will triumph over a limiting belief about those protein bars and how we need them, every time.

The Temporary Inconvenience

Successful people are willing to do the things unsuccessful people will not do.
~ John C. Maxwell.

I will be transparent about this. Nothing worthwhile comes easily and effortlessly. Yes, to shift out of a comfortable, dysfunctional place is going to require some initial discomfort and intentional, dedicated focus every day. Small steps, when consciously and consistently chosen, lead to lasting positive change.

Those who have achieved elevated, sustainable wellness make conscious decisions about what they say yes and no to, based on what supports them. This involves a commitment to personal inquiry and loving openness regarding what food symbolizes in our lives.

I had to go very deep to discover why food was my only—and I mean *only*—source of joy, comfort, and liberation in my life.

Why had I believed food was my only real friend?

If a magic genie could snap her fingers and give you an ideal self as it relates to food and body, what would that look like for you?

And if the genie asked you to get uncomfortable temporarily to foster this ideal self for the rest of your life, would you have the courage to do that?

Before you start second-guessing your capabilities to endure some discomfort, just know that we all have an inner stubborn badass Diva Self who is just waiting to be unleashed and given some damn power. She may be hidden under layers of limiting beliefs about ourselves—thank you, failed diet attempts for fostering this—but she is definitely in you! She is just waiting for you to give her the reins.

I believe that for those of you who have fought yourself with diets, restrictions, and rules, the wisdom of life had you on the journey for a good reason. You learned some hard lessons. For me, it took decades to understand what these lessons were.

I believe that if you are courageous enough to have dieted and restricted your eating, you are courageous enough to be temporarily uncomfortable. That is the only good thing about dieting: It gave us practice to level up our stubborn-girl, headstrong, badassness to fight for something better for ourselves. This may sound contradictory, but our dieting scars are symbols of our inner strengths and wisdom.

You are already resilient, and you have the power.

Now is the time to channel that badassness the right way with the right tools for smart healing. You have the power to reprogram your brain. And the right programming is founded in loving, compassionate inquiry—*not* fighting, depriving, and restricting.

When approached in this manner, our inner resilience works for us in the right ways and grows. And this resilience cannot be purchased with a credit card. It is free and exists in our minds. We become what we think. What we think, we do. It is time to consider what we are really thinking.

Stretching beyond our comfort zones sets us on a pathway to freedom that unleashes personal power we did not know lay within. Diets have toxified our beliefs about our capabilities.

If you can endure a little discomfort now, you can reclaim your inner spirit and take control of living your true life on your terms—your top values are intact, you feel fulfilled, and you no longer feel trapped within yourself.

You can end your war with food.

The Diva in the Driver's Seat

In 2019, the week after Christmas, I was in a typical state for me. As usual, I had binged my way through the holidays, which really meant the previous two months. I was sitting with my 2020 planner, writing my goals, which always started with a weight goal.

I would turn fifty on May 7, 2020, and this would be the year I finally got serious and achieved my best self—by that I meant my ideal size and weight. Never mind other valuable goals, like improving my relationships with family and friends or elevating my career. My weight goal was always at the top of the list because this was my uber-measure of self-worth. I had to achieve this before I could take on anything else.

I wrote out my diet plan, which was a list of restricted foods and those considered more healthful that I would force myself to eat. I'd do weekly weigh-ins on my bathroom scale. I would allow myself some cheating after my weigh-in, which I told myself would be okay because I'd follow up with a hardcore workout to get back on track.

This mode seemed to work for me in my thirties when I was enslaved to the WW regimen. I somehow achieved lifetime membership and my 130-pound champion goal weight with my barbaric tactic of *diet—binge—exercise—repeat*. To me, this was all I knew, and all I believed could ever work for me. I just had to use more willpower, I thought.

I began 2020 as usual: fighting, becoming distracted, feeling uninspired, and slowly giving up by March 1. I coasted until I felt motivated to take up the fight again.

Then COVID-19 struck. Like many others, I was faced with the fear of the unknown. Any sense of control over my life was forced out of my grip. My thriving personal training business halted, and my inner demons shoved their asses into the forefront of my emotional brain. What I thought I had under control turned on me like a boomerang.

On lockdown at home, I devised a rigid plan of controlling my diet. I would start my day with the best of my restrictive food attempts and get in my at-home workout. Then my inner fear-based rebellious beast would take over later in the day, and I would entertain a serious WTF attitude. I began bingeing on Ben & Jerry's ice cream, two pints for dinner every night. This became an uncontrollable pattern that quickly reminded me of the sugar binges that were my escape hatch from pressure in high school. It was all coming back to me at warp speed.

My stomach, head, and emotions were screaming in desperation for relief. My inner child was kicking, screaming, and crying for attention in a bunch of ways. I felt hopeless and desperate. My only solace was the relief the ice cream gave me from all the pain.

Alone with myself and my empty pints of Ben & Jerry's, I finally felt shaken, as if I were a rag doll, and God was telling me it was time for me to face my problem with food. I felt I had to drop my fit pro façade and to get real help. I was on a quest to discover what I had been missing.

My inner wisdom and calling were that I had to admit my powerlessness over my emotional binge eating. I began reading about emotional eating and sugar addiction. I was ready to face my truths and get uncomfortable for freakin' real. I was fed up and exhausted with my inner war and fight.

I was sick and tired of using food, mainly sugar, to relieve myself from some unknown feeling time and time again.

I loved sugar, but it did not love me back. It lied to me. It was killing all aspects of me, and I suddenly felt alive in this truth. I decided to slay the beast instead of letting it slay me. I felt pissed. What had I been missing? I craved freedom and independence from food enslavement in my life like never before.

This pandemic—with respect and acknowledgement of everyone's unique challenges in this crisis—made me truly angry. It brought out my inner resilient badass. I remember watching an episode of *Dr. Phil*, in which he was interviewing women via Zoom and inquiring about their personal challenges during the pandemic. The challenges included fear, alcohol consumption, binge eating, and loss of jobs.

Dr. Phil gave some advice to these women that saved my life and sent me running toward personal development with a surge of openness. He advised them to consider what they could do right now with what was available to them in order to come out stronger and on top of their game when the lockdown was over.

In other words, how could these women look for and act on opportunities to maximize strengths and prepare to come out on top, not deflated and defeated?

That was the inspiration I needed to hear the call to say good-bye to the diet-binge-repeat lifestyle that kept me hijacked and hello to taking on a new pathway of thinking, believing, and acting to help me heal and rewrite my future.

I freakin' wanted more and was willing to do what it took to get it. I became open and curious. I kicked my ego of *knowing it all*—as a fit pro . . . *please!*—or at least thinking I did, to the curb. I hired a personal online health coach who helped me go inward in ways I had never considered. I joined an online community of other wonderful people who shared my struggles with food abuse, dieting, and sugar addiction. Interacting with them daily is what has helped me identify and pulled me through my limiting thoughts. They also gave me belief and courage to write this book.

What did I have to lose?

With the help of my online coach and community, I said a formal goodbye to foods that cause me to feel addicted and hijacked—sugar and flour. I realized they were no longer my friends. I became open to others who were struggling with the similar dieting and emotional binge-eating challenges. I discovered that I was not alone in this shameful war, and I became immersed in the support of this group that gave me the space to share.

With this newfound extensive time to be alone with myself, I inquired what was going on in my head and heart, in relationship to myself. I discovered personal wounds in my life that had been left unhealed. I discovered roots of pain within myself that were prompting me to use food to escape.

I purged my house of all trigger foods, and I programmed my mind with a one-day-at-a-time, don't-break-the-chain mentality to choose whole, unprocessed foods that I enjoyed. I lovingly went inward to rediscover myself as a person. Initially, this was hard. I even cried at times, which felt like I was letting something go. I was also developing a new sense of awareness and connection with myself, which felt newly odd but good.

I felt different—really different. I was healing. I started to feel really good. I felt clean in my head, light in my body, free in my spirit. I was on to something. I was feeling good without abusing food. For the first time ever, I found joy coming from other sources in my life rather than the false beliefs of diets and rebellious bingeing. And, *I never got on the scale*. I just noticed how I felt each day. Thirty days, one at a time, became fifty, then one hundred, and so forth. I have never looked back, only forward. I consider myself a wounded healer, walking a path of forever vigilance for how food makes me feel.

This is my new story. I document my progress from a mind-body-healing perspective, not from a diet strategy. There is no end point, no weigh-in date, and no number on the scale dictating my success. I became my own Diva in the driver's seat of my life.

I found freedom from food, body, and myself for the first time in my life. I realize now that my destiny was to experience and live the war of dieting so that I can understand this at a deep level and help other amazing women like you find their freedom on their terms and never diet again. You can be the Diva in the driver's seat of your life.

I learned to relinquish my rigid thoughts, surrender my control, and become curious about what I could learn from someone else. *I did not know what I did not know.* I began building a toolbox for staying the course with my foods that, as Molly Carmel says in *Breaking Up With Sugar*, loved me back, for real, and for learning how to block the noise of a junk-food society that tries to take me down every day.

The tools in my box are not presented as supplements, bars, or shakes. They come from the mind and heart. Our healing is within that space. Not, remember, with our credit card on Amazon Prime.

BECOME YOUR OWN CEO

I had to push past my judgment of a new way of thinking. Looking for answers in the dark mysterious depths of our minds sounded like something nonsensical and pointless at first—almost *woo-woo.* The fitness-coach part of my personality judged anything emotional or psychological as useless: *Just give me the meal plan and rules that came with the new diet. Never mind all that mindfulness bullshit. All it takes is hard work. Ignore that mental chatter and surge forward! Only tough people who hustle are successful at anything, right?*

The Two Voices Within

Consider the voice you hear in your head who goes with you everywhere. It is like a nagging inner roommate who will not shut up. Some experts estimate that the average number of thoughts per day by an individual is 60,000–80,000.[8] That is a lot of babbling! And those thoughts have a lot of power. They are like the command center of our personal spaceship. The thoughts we have dictate how we feel and how we behave—the quality of our health and spirit.

I continue to struggle with identifying and feeling through that constant chatter in my mind. Part of my healing from toxic dieting involved sitting with this inner chatter and becoming curious about what the noise is. Thoughts in my head are often like a hamster wheel that does not stop. This inner energy has a way of building up and producing feelings of being overwhelmed. That sense can prompt the unwanted habit of using food to escape the pressures of this incessant babbling.

You may be able to separate the chatter into two voices that compete for attention. One is critical, judgmental, tough,

8 Sasson, Remez. "How Many Thoughts Does Your Mind Think in One Hour?" Success Consciousness (blog). successconsciousness.com

and unforgiving. The other is nurturing, loving, kind, and encouraging.

See if you can give faces to the voices inside you by using my personal example. My inner critic's voice is like that of the green-faced Wicked Witch from the *Wizard of Oz*. She took my power and became Captain Bitch of my personal ship for decades. The witch voice would criticize every thought, action, and outcome, telling me I was a failure due to my secret shame of pigging out and lacking willpower. This, sadly, infected my entire character and integrity. The witch beat me down with thoughts that told me that, *as a person*, I was a failure.

Then there is Glinda, the beautiful Witch of the North, who travels in a mystical bubble and wears a sparkling pink gown. She reassures Dorothy that she is safe and capable. Dorothy already has within the power she needs, and she is *enough* just as she is. Glinda represents another voice in my head—my inner, loving coach.

I believe that these two voices have existed in my head for my entire life.

Do voices such as these accompany you throughout your day?

Sadly, the world encourages us to give power to the inner critic voice in our heads over our inner loving coach. Think of how much easier it is to pay attention to inner critic babble than believe the nurturing guidance and love of our inner loving coach. Somehow, we believe that the inner critic will *toughen us up or keep us grounded.*

I believed this and unknowingly gave almost all my power to my inner critic. Rest assured, however, we have tools to help us find the invisible bucket of water to melt her and all that babble. Part of our healing depends on it. It requires much more from us than following a food plan, by the way, but the payoff is well worth the discomfort of filling the inner bucket of water as a tool to melt the voice berating us with criticisms and judgments.

Glinda was soft, kind, and gentle. I believed if I listened to her trying to bring out my feelings and emotions, it would make me weak and vulnerable. I minimized nurturing myself. I developed a self-harming, limiting belief that I didn't need nurturing. I wanted to be tough because I believed only relentlessly tough people were hard workers who became successful in their lives. They were the survivors. I was conditioned to believe soft people got trampled and left behind. This scared me.

Glinda spoke with a softness that made me feel heard and safe. Her voice validated that I was enough, that I would somehow be okay just being me. *There's no place like home. You are enough, Tracy. You have everything you need right here in your heart, and you are capable of great things.*

We have two voices in our heads that, when recognized with openness and curiosity, provide the opportunity to discover an escape from the inner war with food, body, and self. I encourage you now to consider two characters to identify with those two voices inside your emotional mind and the chatter in your head.

To this day I have to work hard at hearing the loving coach and allowing her voice to have power. It means cultivating a kind of vigilance—watching my mind and making choice after choice throughout the conscious hours to turn my attention toward her rather than the Wicked Witch.

This is healing. This is how we choose to move out of the old habits into a new way of thinking, believing, acting, and living. This is how we choose health, again and again.

The Promotion

When considering the two voices that comprise our inner chatter, we develop an awareness within ourselves. We ultimately have a choice when it comes to listening to the inner critic (Wicked Witch) or the inner loving coach (Good Witch).

How in the world do we slow and direct our thoughts and allocate this power in the hamster wheel of our mind?

It is as simple as deciding to fire the wicked-witch inner critic and promote the good-witch inner loving coach.

To face the mental chatter, we must endure the initial, awkward discomfort of sitting quietly and asking: *What do I feel?* If you've been avoiding pain, depression, or anxiety by keeping busy or, as I had always done, by bolting to food as an escape, this stage may feel foreign and unpleasant. This can be a big surprise, and it was for me. I had a few crying meltdowns as I pulled back the layers of onion I had grown to ignore my pain and force myself to be tough. But stick with it; try it for short periods at first—maybe only five minutes at a time.

See if you can inquire with curiosity about the voices and ideas residing in your head. Slowly unravel the dialogue that currently exists. Notice, observe, without judgment. You are taking inventory in this moment, not assessing or qualifying what you hear.

As you listen, you may recognize some of these phrases from the critic:

- *You are not good enough—worthy enough—qualified enough.*
- *You do not fit in.*
- *You don't measure up.*
- *Don't take risks!*
- *Stay small; stay safe.*
- *I need doughnuts!*

The inner critic thrives on ideas such as these. The inner critic builds limiting beliefs that keep us in an emotional prison until we learn to face them, to see them for what they are, to allow them to flow through us, and to release them. These limiting beliefs are typically rooted in past experiences—childhood for example. The more we feel these wounds or scars in our relationship with ourselves, we subconsciously adopt these limiting beliefs as facts.

This mistaken terrain becomes so familiar to us, it becomes a source of comfort, so we cling to it. This, in turn, keeps us stuck. To reframe our thoughts and repattern our minds require of us to move away from the familiar, to move outside our comfort zone with conscious awareness and intention.

The inner loving coach speech on the other hand, says things such as:

- *You are enough just as you are.*
- *You are worthy—you matter—you are valid.*
- *You are resilient.*
- *You are capable.*
- *You are loved and lovable.*
- *You are beautiful.*
- *You are just fine.*
- *We do not really need doughnuts right now.*

The inner loving coach chatter is the opposite of limiting—it is empowering. When we intentionally give power to our inner loving coach talk, we build the belief that we can improve what we choose in our lives—especially, that we can break free from toxic dieting.

It is up to you to decide which voice to promote. It is tempting to keep that Wicked Witch exactly where she is because we have built her a cozy, comfy nest inside our emotional brain. We've subconsciously made her Captain Bitch of our ship for way too long. But one of the keys to permanent weight loss and shifting yourself from the inside out is to decide which voice you listen to.

Think of how your mind works when you begin restricting yourself on a diet plan. Do you have empowering, nurturing thoughts? I know I never did. I always had a fighter mentality, chasing after a dreamy outcome. I felt angry toward others and even had a sense of disliking them. My resentment kept me separate from those around me and kept me in a state of disembodiment from my own self. It's easier to hear the voice of the critic when we feel isolated. We can only heal with love as the foundation. Fighting ourselves will never work, and that is the same with diets—they rarely sustain us.

Understand that our inner world is rooted in the following chain:

Thoughts → Feelings → Attitudes → Actions

We become what we think about over and over. Thoughts become feelings. Feelings become attitude. Attitude directs actions. This pattern clarifies how habits are formed through repetition. Habits essentially become who we are and how we live our lives. Since you are the CEO of yourself, you can decide to give Glinda, your inner loving coach, the promotion and begin to steer your thought patterns toward an elevating chain of command.

Attitude Is Power

We have the power of our minds.

I want to acknowledge that it is so freakin' easy to think like a victim, to feel overwhelmed by a lack of understanding of self or other circumstances in the past that contributed to a mental state of being and relationship with ourselves. The inner wisdom of your food story calls you to be curious and inquisitive.

Positivity is a choice. Deliberately choosing it requires intentional daily practice.

Gratitude or victimhood: which do you choose?

A positive attitude does not magically arise in people who appear on the outside to be consistently uplifting and happy. They are consciously *choosing* to be this way, choosing to give off vibrations of love to the world. While, yes, we all come from different places in our lives with varying circumstances and challenges, we all have the same opportunity to choose positive thoughts over negative thoughts to recalibrate our attitudes, which have more power than we realize.

It sounds so simple, but how can you make it happen?

My son, Jackson Desjardins, is one of the best representatives of choosing to be happy. Jackson is an amazing twenty-four-year-old man who is an online entrepreneur and my partner in our mother-son podcast called The Happy Grind Movement https://podcasts.apple.com/us/podcast/the-happy-grind-movement/id1610179107. He takes pride in his daily intention of spreading good cheer and joy to anyone and everyone he encounters. He delights in saying hello with generous enthusiasm. It often shifts people's energy from *blah* to *awesome* simply by smiling, saying hello, and appreciating people in an authentic way.

Jackson chooses a positive attitude, even on his challenging days. It has become part of his daily mental programming. This is his daily intention, as programmed by his inner CEO in command, and he relies on it to maintain a positive mindset. As a result, he is the happiest and most self-disciplined person I know. I've heard comments from others who feel the same way. He is regularly thanked for making other people's days. His behavior is a model for me and reminds me to keep my own shit together and always look for the good.

Allow me to emphasize here that this is a conscious choice he makes each day, and he does not take it for granted. He is proof that we can program our minds to be who we want to be, starting with our thoughts.

When you wake in the morning and start your day, you can choose which thoughts you focus on. These thoughts will dictate your attitude. That attitude then contributes to the actions and behaviors you choose for your day.

Will the actions and behaviors you choose support you or bring you down?

My attitude determines whether I see the world for the good or the ugly. I have noticed this integrates with my food story. When I consciously seek the good in circumstances and people, my craving for junk food practically disappears. My spirit feels nurtured and healthy. This is a choice. This does not happen automatically; also, friends, it has taken me more than thirty-five years to practice, and it is ongoing. Believe me, not all days are sunshine and rainbows, despite my best intentions set in the morning. Let's get real about this.

In fact, as I write this chapter, this particular week has been an emotional roller coaster of challenges for me both personally and professionally. The difference is that I no longer use food to distract or comfort myself. I simply inquire as to how I am feeling and what I really need in that moment. I practice bringing in the inner loving coach as CEO and quieting the inner critic. *Tracy, you already have the power within you to protect yourself.* Thank you, Glinda.

What I think becomes how I feel.

How I feel becomes my attitude for the day.

My attitude for the day determines my actions: do I eat healthful, tasty food that I like and that supports me, nourishes me, and makes me feel amazing, or do I distract, punish, and sabotage myself with doughnuts and ice cream?

I choose to tell myself uplifting, nurturing things; I note examples of loving kindness, and I look for what it is good in any given moment in my day. This practice is my shield, my suit of armor, to navigate through continual triggers that could derail my choice. I'll say again that this is a conscious practice—it is not my default way of being, not even after all this time. One must commit oneself over and over, each day, in small and big ways, to change.

1. Name three things, right now, that you are grateful for. You've likely heard this before. But have you *done it?*

2. Repeat this tomorrow and the next day. Practice makes better, even on those crappy days!

3. Notice how this over time creates a chain—each time you do it creates a new link in your chain of positive thought. This will slowly build your inner suit of armor to protect your chosen focus: the good in you and in the world.

Whoever thought that, simply by taking 100 percent responsibility for shifting your thoughts, you could create a secret pathway to weight loss and life improvements?!

There are more tools to come for you, but please commit to developing your suit of armor by increasing your awareness of what you are thinking. You are going to need this before all else. Get comfy and rein in the power of your thoughts. No victim. No cynicism. No bullshit. This is mandatory. Onward!

CHAPTER FOUR

A Powerful Trifecta

Ultimately, we all want answers for our unwanted eating concerns. We want solutions we can rely on to support us in living an abundant life. I call this the *Path of Excellence* for food, body, and self. We desire an end to routine of starting over with another diet plan, hoping we'll finally get our shit together, lose unwanted weight, and sustain an eating plan so we can free up mental space to live a purposeful life. We are all worthy of achieving this.

I believe the diet industry places way too much profit-driven emphasis on the food and body aspects of wellness.

Just eat clean and exercise, right?

We are all sick of hearing that.

The truth is, healing a challenged relationship with food, body, and self involves a trifecta of focus. It is definitely *not* all about food and exercise. Believe me, if it were, I would have had success with this a long time ago. Here is where we begin to create your very own Path of Excellence.

MIND	+	BODY	+	SPIRIT
(our emotions)	+	(food & movement)	+	(inner hearts & being)

=HEALING
= (from the inside out)

You can create your very own toolbox for achieving long-lasting results and inner peace, perhaps for the first time ever! This toolbox is your customized collection of strategies for your Path of Excellence. There is no one-size-fits-all solution. Once you discover these tools and put them into use, you release yourself from the war within, and you experience freedom like never before.

Self-trust will be yours, as well as abundance in your life. Oh, and by the way, those unwanted pounds of bodyfat will melt off the right way—with your toolbox in action. Let's get working!

MIND AND EMOTION

The pathway to truly breaking free from the shackles of dieting and finding true peace begins with understanding our mindset. We must develop the ability to clearly identify feelings and emotions. Dieting focuses on food plans and rules, but it rarely addresses *how to think and feel* in a holistic manner that serves us. Healing from toxic dieting and shedding unwanted pounds and body fat must start with programming a supportive, and attentive, mindset. This mindset programming will become a tool for staying the course and send you down that chute of turning to food to ignore yourself. It will keep you on track even when all of society around you is trying to derail you.

Most dieting programs do not encourage going inward and being aware of how we are thinking and feeling. The emphasis is typically placed on the food plans and associated food goals. This robs us of understanding what our appetite and inner wisdom are trying to tell us. When we learn to connect with our feelings and emotions before emphasizing food strategies at any given time, with the guiding, patient voice coming from our inner loving coach as CEO, we then open the space to be curious about how to meet our needs in any given moment. The key here is learning how to become self-aware of feelings and emotions within our minds.

Developing Self-awareness

I had missed out on how to identify feelings and emotions for most of my life. I was afraid of feeling, afraid of emotions. I had no idea where my feelings—mainly the unpleasant ones—were coming from. I just felt constant chatter in my head. In my quest to be tough and strong, I believed it was unsafe to show any vulnerability because then, I would appear weak.

When we learn to feel, we begin to heal the interior tug-of-war regarding food, body, and self. Many of us were taught that feelings and emotions were to be ignored and minimized. But the opposite is true. Feelings and emotions are powerful clues and guideposts as to what we need at any given moment. And most of the time, friends, what we need is *not* food. Boy, did I ever get that wrong!

How do we develop self-awareness? This can be quite challenging for those of us who have been surging through our lives on autopilot, but it is rather simple and is the ticket for discovering how to meet your needs and, honestly, take the best care of yourself—because only *you* can do that.

Stop.

Breathe deeply in and out a few times. Find calm in your mind. Go inward and find your inner loving coach voice. In whatever situation you are at the time, and whatever is going on, you can access your inner CEO to talk gently to you and begin asking simple questions, as you would when speaking to a child:

- *What is going on here?*
- *What are you feeling?*
- *It's okay to feel this way. Let's just sit with this feeling for a while and allow it to just be there. We are going to be fine.*

We are going somewhere with this, as we pave the road for Step Three, but first, let's dive a bit deeper and move from self-awareness and learning to identify feelings to understanding emotions and how they relate to our food challenges.

Understanding Emotional Eating

In Chapter One, we referenced the concepts of food and love as well as emotional hunger. If we recognize how we, as infants, associate food as a direct source of love and comfort, we can then understand how we can be programmed to escape to food for immediate relief from uncomfortable feelings and emotional states. Many of us, myself included, have developed this habit subconsciously and feel overpowered by this instinctive action of bolting to food to soothe, numb, distract, or simply to fill a void that we seem powerless to control.

Restrictive dieting can fuel emotional eating challenges because it focuses on logical food programming and rules. This signals us to ignore the innate signals relating to our appetite that come from our feelings and emotions. We believe that we should ignore our own intuition and trust the rules of the diet to sustain us. This usually fuels the restricted rebel inside our emotional mind which can unleash an emotional binge-eating monster from within that intensifies an additional problem with food, body, and self.

Learning how to become mindful of our feelings and emotional states at any given moment is a critical element in healing a damaged relationship with food, building self-trust, and repairing our wounds. We begin to understand how easy it is to use food to escape from what our spirit is telling us we really need. Be willing to go inward and inquire as to what you are really hungry for.

If you have struggled with using food to cope with emotional needs as I have, consider what other things besides food bring you joy, relief, pleasure, soothing comfort, or escape. Take a moment to ponder this question and jot your answers down in your journal or document it where you have written your food story.

I had the realization that, most of the time, when I was bolting to food for relief of something, what I really needed was a time-out and mental break from my over-packed daily schedule. I was trying to use sugary junk foods for instant energy. I now take 10-minute power naps as needed or walk my dogs to clear my head and recalibrate with a peaceful activity. And it works!

What situations or circumstances do you face that prompt uncomfortable emotions where you may find yourself using food to fill voids?

Taking time to reflect on this and on new ways to nurture yourself during those times are powerful acts of healing self-care and learning to self-regulate.

Developing New Coaching Skills

Reprogramming your mindset with an inner loving coach voice is free. It is your most powerful tool. This starts with curiosity about feelings and being open to exploring solutions to soothe all your emotions without abusing food.

In Chapter One, we learned how appetite is a hunger within that is calling for attention. We also learned about physical and emotional hunger and the complexity of these concepts. For the chronic dieter, the feeling of any form of hunger, whether physical or emotional, can feel like a tsunami from within.

What are the hungers we believe food can satisfy?

- We all hunger for our place in the world from which we give and receive love in one form or another.
- We all hunger to feel good enough to share joy in our own unique ways.
- We all hunger for our identity and the confirmation that we belong.

Life gets complicated by problems. We all know this. It can be way too easy to bolt to that reliable source of immediate relief: food.

I did that for decades. If only I had known how to stop in that moment and ask myself what I was truly hungry for. *What is eating at me*, rather than *what am I eating?* Diet culture does nothing to promote healthy emotional connection with one's true hunger. It focuses on food rules, restriction, and deprivation and feeds our inner rebel and sells us on the insanity of its particular game. And it always fails *us*, but the industry itself swims in profits.

When we meet ourselves with loving curiosity and inquiry, solutions for self-care arise. We allow the wisdom of life to direct us toward our own healing. This increases our tolerance for unpleasant circumstances, feelings, and emotions in an empowering new way. We learn to ask ourselves questions that help us be patient with ourselves; thereby, we strengthen our resolve to meet our needs authentically. This is our guidepost within our spirit.

Your new CEO of self, your inner loving coach, is now helping you program your inner software or mindset from a place of love and compassion, not only for yourself but also extending that to others. See if you notice whether the little things in life that used to set you off no longer have that power. Inner peace provides a beacon toward wise healing. We truly can develop an inner environment in our headspace. We can gather a box of strategic tools to help us when our lives go batty, which is pretty often—sometimes daily.

When the sneaky callings urge us to use food to numb, escape, and abandon our mission for healing—and they will—we are ready with our inner tools. Without them, we are helpless.

STEP THREE: Commit to Daily Personal Inquiry and Master Your Self-Awareness

1. Stop, in your mind—wherever you are and whatever is going on.

2. Take a few slow, deep breaths.

3. Ask yourself:

   What am I feeling (emotion)?
   What do I really need?
   What will I do right now?

Keep in mind that no healing happens overnight. We cannot click a few buttons to order our online recovery after decades of dieting failures and frustrations. We cannot instantly undo the damage done both psychologically and physically. The only way we can heal is to start with tiny steps. This is not the time for setting a deadline or tracking weight. It is time to reframe our thoughts, emotions, and feelings.

We are simply on the road now—on the healing journey, taking one step at a time, one day at a time, every day. The process will yield sustainable, lasting recovery that will unleash space in which you can begin living your purposeful life. Essentially, these small, consistent steps are all you need to release the inner shackles of dieting and fighting yourself.

FOOD AND BODY

So far, we have worked with mind and emotions, getting to the roots of how our mental chatter can be our worst enemy. We now understand that through Step Three and personal inquiry, self-love, and activating our inner loving coaching voice, day by day, we form strong foundations for the next component of healing.

Of course as an experienced, jaded, and recovered dieter, I know that this is the part you are all waiting for, right? You're ready for the food plan.

But there is no food plan in this book. Instead, I am going to teach you how to develop your own. What you choose to eat is none of my business. And frankly, it's no one else's either.

Who the hell would I be, telling you what to eat?

I will not set you up for unleashing your inner rebel to work against you—that is what diets do. I am simply going to get real about how *you* can decide what foods serve you best. And it is crazy simple. I am going to give you the badass truth, and you can take it and run with it on your terms. No rules, no regulations, and a big *hell no!* to weighing yourself as the gold standard measure of success.

Our dieting drama and ongoing battleground of dysfunctional eating habits can leave us malnourished in many ways, such as:

- Hormonal imbalances
- Macronutrient imbalances
- Brain chemistry imbalances
- Food allergies
- Food addictions
- Sugar addictions
- Gut and digestive challenges
- Disruptive sleep patterns

Shifting our food choices from mostly processed and tongue-indulgent foods toward whole and unprocessed, truly nourishing foods takes patience, persistence, willingness, dedication, and a strong commitment to your Personal Powerful Why or PPW (see Chapter Three to refresh your memory about PPW).

Time to Clean Up!

When my kids were little, I'd tell them it was time to clean up the playroom—a disaster zone of toys, games, VHS tapes, and other junk. It looked like a hedonistic war zone in that room most of the time, just utter chaos. *Clean up* meant all toys were put back in the appropriate tubs and bins, and the room looked orderly. This provided us all a sense of peace, calm, structure, and refreshment to our living space.

How does this relate to the mind and body?

The content and quality of what we have been eating and drinking for decades has taken up chaotic space in our bodies and brains, appearing in symptoms such as excess fat, extra pounds, inflammation, brain fog, and low energy.

How do we get control of our interior chaotic mess?

By conducting a Cleanup from within that will make us feel recharged, refreshed, and rebooted. I am not a dietician, nutritionist, medical practitioner, or anyone who has any business telling *you* what to eat. I will even go as far as to ask you to ponder if you really believe that you need one of those professionals telling you what to eat.

Has that worked for you in the past?

I gather not, or else you would not have picked up this book. You are a unique spirit on a unique pathway. You hold within you the authentic answers for how to arrive at your best self regarding food and body. You have your own answers about the *what*, the *why*, and the *how* for foods. If this frustrates you, I completely understand.

We traded in our self-trust and common sense the minute we bought in to our first diet.

As mentioned previously, diets focus on the perfect food plans and rules. In reality—and I speak from experience here, friend—any of these plans do work *if followed precisely*. I know that's a shock to read after everything I've said so far.

What can I possibly mean?

The problem is that diets are typically *not sustainable.* So dieting is a big game that never ends well. Even if we achieve our *goal weight*, a term I hate, we are left with a sense of panic and desperation.

With traditional diets, once we've achieved that hard-earned goal, we're left wondering what to do. We've fought to get there with tools that resonated with us. We feel like caged tigers after living within someone else's boundaries for a while, and before too long, we slide back to our old ways of eating—or worse—bingeing in reaction to the restriction and deprivation.

As a fitness professional of more than thirty years, I can honestly say that I have yet to meet one single person who started a diet program, achieved their goal weight, and maintained their goal weight while staying on that particular diet—myself included, pals. I have seen many people, including myself, whittle down to even less than their goal weight on a diet, stay there for a brief time, and return to their original size *or more* once they had released themselves from the confines of the restrictive eating.

Clearly, dieting works *temporarily.* But who wants to play Chutes & Ladders with food, body, and sanity for the rest of their life? This diet game is more like a battlefield, not only emotionally, but also biologically and chemically.

The Standard American Diet (SAD) is laden with processed ingredients, additives, chemicals, fat, salt, and sugar. Let's be real, here—this food tastes *great*. It should. The food industry has invested big bucks for scientific research to create the perfect brain-hijacking *bliss point* that turns taste buds and brains into tantrumming, bratty children, demanding more.

Can you eat just one potato chip, french fry, doughnut hole, or Oreo?

We all know the painful dissatisfaction of eating a salad or a juicy apple on day one of a diet after bingeing on junk foods for so long. Our tongues reject this taste because our palate has been rewired for sugar, salt, fat, and the other crap. We have trained ourselves away from natural food. Keep in mind, while our tongues are saying no, our brains are saying: *Yes, please help me!*

There is also the façade of artificial sweeteners and diet foods. I remember feeling addicted to diet sodas. It was like a force from within. I could not go one day without them. Diet foods and diet products create a boomerang effect in our brain, resulting in cravings from hell. Our brains confuse artificial with the real thing. I remember overloading on Fiber One snack bars and other commercial diet-snacky-treat-bars with those sugar alcohols. I was then forced to stay in my home on lockdown for the rest of the night with enough bloat and gas to damn near set my house on fire.

To elevate our lives is to elevate our food choices to those that truly nourish our body and mind. Remember, as Marc

David of the Institute for the Psychology of Eating says: *How we do food is how we do life.*

Do you want a processed-junk life or a fresh, naturally abundant, high-quality life?

Think of the example of putting the highest quality gas in your car versus the cheapest gas. How does your car run?

We must, I repeat, *must* break free from the habitual use of processed foods, junk foods, snack foods, diet junk foods, and foods you believe you *need to keep* for some reason. You know your truth, here, protein-bar peeps. Here is your calling.

STEP FOUR: Perform Your 14-Day Whole-Foods Clean-up Experiment

PART A: This step is to clean up the brain, tongue, and body to give yourself 14 days to consume whole, natural, unprocessed foods as an experiment. How do they make you feel from the inside out—mentally and physically? Give yourself the gift of discovering what nutritional self-care feels like for you.

This is non-negotiable for cleaning up the chemistry in the brain, resetting the tongue and palate, taming the inner child within, and harnessing your power to want nourishing foods. Consider this a personal power washing, from the inside out.

Do not make this complicated. Your common sense knows what processed junk foods are. Do not short-change yourself by thinking you need a diet plan to follow. I encourage you to decide what whole, unprocessed foods you want to eat, so that you can begin designing your own nutritional library of foods that sustain, support, and satisfy you.

Choose your favorites from these suggested categories, and of course, honor your individual food sensitivities or allergies:

- Vegetables and Fruits
- Whole Grains
- Lean meats, fish, and dairy
- Healthy fats, like nuts and avocado and olive oils
- Water

As for condiments? Choose low-salt and low-sugar options and use common-sense amounts.

You may be wondering about portions, which would make sense, since diets have us weighing, measuring, and counting, which can be exhausting.

When we choose whole, natural foods, they help balance the body. Our body will signal when we have had enough and is satiated. If we are eating slowly, and are aware, we can begin to trust our appetite to regulate normally. Remember, we typically do not overeat or binge on apples or salad. We are growing in awareness not only regarding our thoughts and feelings, but also with our inner, natural appetite that regulates once we keep processed, palate-driven, addictive foods off the tongue.

Drink water, my friends. This is non-negotiable. If you do not like water, I will argue that this is when you must make a badass decision to *try harder*. Add a squeeze of a lemon or other citrus fruit. No bubbles, please—that is another crutch that will keep you dreaming of soda.

Consider your pace while eating your meals and snacks. Slow eating provides the opportunity to be present with your food and to experience savoring the abundant taste of whole, natural foods. Slow down and enjoy your bounty of choice and be mindful of *how you are feeling* while you are eating.

I encourage you to wipe the slate clean in all that you currently know about dieting and your past. Adopt a fresh mentality that your new friendship with your food is budding. It will take time to rewire your mind to shift the relationship with food into a place of joy. This joy is expressed by how your food choices love you back and sustain your health instead of inflaming your mind and body, causing erratic cravings and sabotaging you.

In the Cleanup, you learn to nourish yourself from the inside out with foods that you like and *taste good*. I am not asking you to remove the joy in eating. It should *never* feel like that. If it does, something is off. You may have become too restrictive. This is tough, of course, in the Cleanup phase, when we are mentally and physically departing from processed garbage while power washing the brain and palate. They are both accustomed to the dopamine hit from junk and foods designed to target the bliss point. To shun those foods suddenly is like sending a child to boot camp.

When you commit to this experiment—one day at a time, one choice at a time—notice what is happening:

- Are you feeling better focus?
- Improved energy?
- Are you sleeping better?
- How does your belly feel?
- Are you experiencing a new sense of calm?
- Be aware.

You will want more of this feeling, and you will persist, for another day, and another. This builds, and so does your belief in yourself. You are teaching yourself that you can harness your health without being miserable on a diet. You are creating your very own clean, wholesome food library, on your terms, based on foods that love and nourish you, not break you down.

With a one-day-at-a-time focus, we elevate our child, who wants what she wants when she wants it, to our intelligent adult inner loving coach. Despite all the advertising for a quick-fix solution, you know there is no sustainable quick-fix solution to elevating health and lasting weight loss. The solution is found in the balance of mind, body, spirit, and health your way, with your inner wisdom and personalized tools.

Small, repeated choices are what it's all about at this point. You will build a string of successes, one decision at a time, one triumph at a time. The little wins will each contribute to the grand prize of improved health, energy, and outlook.

Friends, do not confuse your Cleanup with a diet. Here are the differences and the benefits:

1. A Cleanup is like performing a factory reset to your brain and body. I believe that unless we wipe it clean with powerful super-agents, like clean food, and stop putting in all—and I mean *all*—anti-foods and artificial junk, we will stay hijacked and addicted to chemicals and sugar.

2. A Cleanup pushes past the nonsense, giving your brain and body a freakin' chance to breathe and restart and not be controlled by internal liars. You are giving yourself a chance to experience what it is like to not have cravings for junk anymore and to feel truly nourished, clean, and focused, perhaps for the first time ever. The first few days are the most difficult, as the body is detoxing from the inside out. Typical symptoms include headache, fogginess, and fatigue. But stay the course, because this is temporary, and there is powerful, refreshing space on the other side, where you begin to taste true wellness.

Ensure you give yourself loving space for your Cleanup. This is not an experiment that is tacked onto a crazy-busy time in your life. Give yourself time for relaxing activities that you enjoy and extra sleep. Remember, we are talking about cultivating self-love, which also means self-care.

After the fourteen days of serious Cleanup dedication, you will experience the wonderful benefits of eating whole foods, such as:

- Decreased inflammation
- Decreased or eliminated cravings
- Improved mental concentration
- Better sleep
- Increased energy
- Decreased bloating

After eating this way *and allowing yourself to notice changes*, you will have a stronger sense of the power of food as medicine to support you, not to sabotage you with the empty promise of a hedonistic escape. As you progress on the 14-Day Whole-Foods Cleanup, you understand and experience the magic of true nourishment from whole foods. The abundance of vitamins and minerals clean the unwanted inflammatory intruders in your brain and body. And now you are tasting what it feels like to be in your body while it is thriving on nutritional medicine.

The Path of Excellence

So, you've made it through the 14-Day Whole-Foods Cleanup Experiment—*what happens now?*

Remember, we are not talking about dieting here. We are talking about noticing the results of this experimental rebooting of your brain and body from the inside out. This is the new reality, guided by your common sense. Taste what it feels like to *be healthy* and vibrant. What happens now is you sustain this new lifestyle on your terms, expanding your nutritional choices within the realm of clean eating.

It is time to design your Path of Excellence. It is paved with whole, unprocessed, clean foods *whose taste you enjoy*, foods that love and support you. Over the last fourteen days, you've built up a library of foods that you can rely on to make you feel healthy and amazing.

Learn to shop and prepare these foods in ways that appeal to you. See Chapter Five for a detailed outline of how you can do this. Learn how to choose restaurants and take-out places that offer these foods on their menu. Those places *do* exist. I eat out quite a bit and have figured out where to go and how to stay focused in all types of restaurants. It just takes commitment and focus.

Because I know how what I chew and swallow will make me feel, I easily stay dedicated to wanting vibrancy versus my old ways. I am no longer willing to trade wellness for a quick hit of junk food dopamine. Key here is the *feeling*—learning to recognize and appreciate the feeling of good food doing good for my body, mind, and spirit. I enlist *feeling* to guide my choices for what is *good food*.

Learning the art of eating to satiation, not to the point of being stuffed, is a habit that can naturally evolve when we choose whole foods. I never, ever remember a time when I binged on apples, carrots, or roasted chicken. When we choose whole, unprocessed foods, our appetites cooperate because we are becoming truly nourished.

Relax in knowing that there is no one cookie-cutter, one-size-fits-all perfect diet. Period. We are all biological individuals when calculating our nutritional best, and that is part of what makes us unique and amazing human beings. Your job is to be patient enough with yourself to find the right balance of whole foods that truly support you from the inside out and provide a reliable, sustainable, foundation for you to live your life to the fullest.

Walking the Path of Excellence, you develop confidence and trust in your food programming and can live your life without berating yourself. There is no failure because you ate sugary, starchy foods on vacation or at a fancy event because there is no diet to break. Our goal is to find a balanced plan that sustains us in feeling truly nourished, not restricted, depleted, and exhausted.

When I adopted a super-simple approach to my food choices, a rainbow of relief and freedom arose. As I began nourishing my body, mind, and palate with whole foods *that I liked*—don't give me celery or mushrooms!—guess what else happened? My body released any excess fat and pounds that it was holding on to that my blueprint finally revealed it did not need.

I ended up in a size of clothing that I never dreamed I would naturally fit into. And here is the big deal: I am not the slightest bit panicked about *keeping the weight off* because I have finally, for the first time ever, found a way to eat holistically that I can do anywhere, anytime, and sustain forever.

Here is your super crazy simple game plan. This is how you design your Path of Excellence, moving forward with your new relationship with food:

- Clean up from the inside out. Choose whole foods that have not been modified commercially.
- Make friends with foods that are true to your greater good, based on your experiment with *how you feel* when you eat them.
- Choose the whole, natural, unprocessed foods you enjoy, which have proven to love you back by making you feel satisfied and vibrant, and which support you in building your best self.
- Finally, keep exploring more whole foods to add to your library.

And now, you walk this Path of Excellence, one day at a time, in a loving personal experiment with your chosen foods and how your body feels when digesting them. If this sounds frustrating and daunting, please understand, that is your inner critic stomping its feet and attempting to pull you back to the land of quick-fixes and childlike tantrums. Acknowledge it, thank it for alerting you to the fact that you're doing something different, and tell it to go sit in the corner.

The 80/20 Idea

Here we come to the big question: *What about my old favorites and treats?*

This is when—with uber loving consideration, self-awareness, and your inner loving coach at the helm—*you* decide how and when you will integrate treats back into your life. The 80/20 idea refers to the proportion of mindful, whole-foods eating—80 percent of the time—to the 20 percent of time when you can choose to enjoy some of your favorite treat-like foods on your own terms, in appropriate portions. In this way, you are less likely to feel restricted during holidays, celebrations, and special events.

The 80/20 idea is key to wielding your power of choice and negotiation on your terms. Because I've come from a background of serious sugar sensitivity, I have developed a heightened self-awareness how I view treats in my life—which is with caution, intention, and vigilance. I know how amazing I feel when I keep sugar off my Path of Excellence.

I also know that my life involves special occasions on which I might want to test the waters with sugar.

The 20 percent is made up of your indulgences, on your terms. These are not lapses or mistakes—they are planned, never bolted to. Think of special occasions in which you plan to savor your 20 percent. This is easier than you think: Remember the cleanup foods you chose from the chart earlier in this chapter? Those are the baseline Best Diva foods for your regular consumption. Once you have identified those foods, they become your food besties.

Here is a secret I learned with clarity for my 80/20: I took out my twelve-month calendar—I am a paper-and-pencil kind of Diva—and put stars on all the days that are special to me. I starred all holidays, birthdays, and other special occasions and vacation days. I divided that total number by 365 days in the year. This totaled less than 20 percent of my life in that given year to enjoy my treats. I was so excited to see this. I felt this clarity provided me with confidence and self-trust that I was not deprived of my favorite indulgences. I had planned for these. Suddenly, my risk for weekend cheat days, which were always binges, did not exist anymore.

I was designing my life as it related to food. My inner loving coach explained to me the power of delayed gratification, which is code for *badass self-discipline*. This discipline makes sense to me; it's on my terms, with no dieting. Nothing is off limits. I plan for my indulgences; I am not freefalling. I am careful to keep my inner rebellious child in her place.

Over time, I have learned I can *savor* these celebratory foods—I can eat them slowly, taste them, and enjoy them, guilt-free. I no longer feel like I need huge portions of cake and ice cream or sneak more when no one is looking. Nor do I feel a drive to sabotage myself by rebelling against a diet. I have learned to coach myself lovingly. I know I nourish myself each day with foods that are medicinal, whole, and natural. I eat these foods for good reasons that support my Personal Powerful Why, which is always front and center. I eat consciously in a way that doesn't promote cravings or feelings of deprivation from sugar or junk.

You, too, can choose your foods based on how you know real food makes you feel—amazing. The ticket for living an abundant life is having energy, vibrancy, and good health. You can do this, my friends. This is how you figure it out for yourself on your terms. Once you release the addictive shackles of processed food consumption and reset your brain and palate with nature's bounty, you gain clarity and, as a result, shed unwanted body fat and pounds.

Cheat Day Only Cheats Yourself

I used to make the dieting mistake of a cheat day on the weekends. That never worked for me because I had the deprivation mentality all week long. I was also consuming artificial sweeteners out the wazoo, which prompted beast-like cravings. I would binge like a monster on Saturday, usually Sunday too, and start over on Monday in a bad place. For this reason, I do not recommend cheat days on weekends.

First of all, this suggests a negative association—*cheat* is an ugly word. We are no longer cheating on ourselves because we are not on diets. We are choosing to live our lives on purpose, walking our Path of Excellence. With our customized whole-food design, we know that we could have whatever we want to eat at any time, but we are *choosing* foods that elevate us from the inside out 80 percent of the time. We also know that our 20 percent is planned, and we have reined in delayed gratification like a champ by now.

With our inner loving coach helping us through heavy emotional days and stressful situations with personal inquiry (review **Step Three** in Chapter Three), we now trust ourselves to not fall prey to junk foods for relief from life's sucker punches and inescapable chaos.

For further customized support, I recommend seeking a holistic doctor or naturopath who can assist with individualized testing for food allergies, sensitivities, digestive challenges, vitamin deficiencies, hormone levels, and other concerns you may have. This is not required, but it is a good idea to get a baseline for any way you might improve your nutrition. When we clean up the brain with nutritional medicine, the cravings for processed foods, salt, and sugar subside and even go away.

When you notice how true wellness feels in your body, you want more wellness because it feels right. You may have never felt anything like these before. It takes a willingness to stay the course with your whole foods and give yourself a chance to experience this.

What is the alternative?

To stay right where you are and keep fighting yourself over cravings and restrictive, on-and-off diet plans.

They never supported you over the long haul in the past, so why would that change for you now?

This is the pathway of your discovery of the foods that are suitable for your library of healing and delicious choices. Adopt an anti-diet strategy now.

Move Your Body

Our physical bodies crave the other part of physical wellness: movement. Friends, this is nonnegotiable. We all know the truth that exercise provides immense benefits to our physical bodies, including prevention of numerous diseases. There are also many psychological benefits of exercise that can help ease symptoms of depression and anxiety.

General recommendations for exercise include thirty minutes per day of moderate physical activity, whether in one session or broken up into segments throughout the day.[9]

How simple is this?!

If a thirty-minute brisk walk is too much to start with all at once, you can do three ten-minute walks per day. Of course, there are next-level options to build upon this, but let's start simply, with thirty minutes of moderate movement per day. When we start simply, we give ourselves the loving chance to celebrate accomplishment one day at a time. This builds our confidence and strength, inside and out.

Let's check in on the emotions here for a moment. Exercise can be a dauting, scary prospect for many people. It can trigger feelings of dread, inadequacy, embarrassment, failure, fear, perceived pain, and more. Based on past experiences and associations with exercise, we can all develop limiting beliefs about what exercise means to us.

I used to believe I failed at several sports as a younger person, despite my efforts. But now I see that I tried, and that effort is a success in itself, regardless of talent or ability. My perceived failure, however, later led me to the understanding that I did not need to be an athlete. I discovered the power of exercise and aerobic activity in my own way—a way that loved me back and spoke to my soul: group fitness classes.

---

9 mayoclinic.org

I felt the first pangs of love for this kind of movement back in my childhood. My dad encouraged me as a small child to run around to loud oldies music in our basement while he exercised. I totally loved just sweating to oldies. It was a blast and felt great. When I was an early teen, he took me with him to the local health club. I discovered this amazing new experience that was all the rage—aerobics class.

As the youngest participant, my free spirit came out of hiding temporarily. I jumped around to eighties music with other smiling people of all shapes and sizes. The class was led by a strong, badass instructor who was not the skinny norm, but was a strong, fit, happy, magnetic force of inspiration to the class.

As I got older, I attended classes by myself. One day, a friendly new instructor I admired immensely, Lisa, called me up to the front of the class and gave me a shot at teaching the group. The song was "Danger Zone." I went crazy with enthusiasm. We did jumping-jacks, high kicks, and in-place jogging all to the beat of the loud music. We all shouted out together in celebration. I thought: *This is living!*

I felt as if I were back in fourth grade but stuffed in my leotard this time and bringing joy, being my zany, unapologetic self. There was no competition. No judgment. People smiled, laughed, and sweated together with loud music, wearing crazy outfits and creating *magical* energy, collectively. We were sharing a zest for life, and this became my new escape from the pressures of my troubled self.

I consistently felt awesome after every aerobics class I took. I was onto something here. I felt like this was saving my life in some way, and now I see it was.

My true spirit was unleashed and alive again. This was my therapy from feeling like a fat girl with no talents, gifts, or identity. I found my happy place in that aerobics room with those wonderful people of all sizes and shapes and that instructor who believed in me. I began attending my aerobics classes regularly between my dieting attempts and binge-eating episodes. I noticed that exercise just made me feel better.

Find a way to move your body that you enjoy, and schedule thirty minutes per day to do it. I challenge anyone claiming they do not have time for movement to consider their mindset and excuses. Then, envision being forced to make time for declining health lifestyle modifications that will be required in your future if you ignore your body's natural craving for movement.

Movement offers us:

- Physical and mental health
- Vitality
- Freedom and independence

Which all leads to living your Best Diva Life!

After all my experience working in fitness, I shout the following statement from the rooftops after countless personal failures—which are actually valuable lessons learned—and observations in the fitness industry:

Exercise is a supplement to nutrition
for healing and nourishing the body
from the inside out.

SPIRIT AND INNER QUEEN

In the musical *Grease*, good-girl protagonist Sandy Olsson is watching the rest of the gang from afar and reflecting on her identity and values. In a reprise of "Look at Me, I'm Sandra Dee," she sings that it's time to take a deep breath and say *goodbye, Sandra Dee*. She decides to break out of her comfort zone and face her fear of putting herself forward in a new scary, but exciting, way.

During a period in my life, I said good-bye to my Tracy Lee—kind of funny how it rhymes with the show tune. I had spent most of my life guarding and fighting something that left me stuck in a Princess-like, wishful mode. I needed everybody else's approval. My free spirit had gone dormant and was ignored, and I was just trying to be somebody that I was not.

I learned I could rewrite my story, think about who I was meant to be and what I really wanted to do with my life.

My life had more substance than starting over on a diet every Monday. I felt something shifting—my inner Queen was emerging, and I was finally beginning to trust that I am enough, and I can live my life in my Path of Excellence on my terms and achieve the best version of my real self.

I did not give a rat's ass anymore if I had external approval from the world. This is the best gift of all: liberation.

The Power of Presence

When we turn away from the diet mentality, we tap in to our spirit who *knows* what is best for us. We connect with our inner loving coach, feel our feelings, understand the true nature of our cravings, and allow the calling of *wisdom* to guide us. We desire a shift in our reality—for substance, for truth. Essentially, we learn the power of presence.

This is tapping in to the archetype of our Queen. She is mature; she stands tall with grace and wisdom. The Queen is ready to block out the incessant, nonsensical noise and chaos of the diet industry and is ready to *figure this shit out*. The Queen leads your quest for how to eat for nourishment, health, and well-being, so you can freakin' get on with your life and rock on with your Best Diva Self. She believes in being well as the path to discovering your God-given life's purpose and then doing it. She trusts. She knows. She is empowered.

Approaching healing as the Queen, we appreciate common sense from a state of presence and calm. We view choices through the mature perspective that we are ready to eat for true nourishment because health feels great. All of a sudden, we feel confident. We feel empowered to begin living for ourselves, not dying in desperation for outside approval. What the world thinks of us is irrelevant. We love ourselves as we are and can spot the commercialized, diet-marketing bullshit immediately from within our confident Queen.

This is true freedom and liberation as a healthy, vibrant, mature woman.

Satisfying Spiritual Hunger

Obsessing about food and our bodies has sucked the life out of our souls. Our job is to step up and take on a journey of healing from within—an expedition of self-inquiry, like a treasure hunt to find gems that make us unique and magnificent people who are alive on Earth to contribute with purpose and passion. The purpose and passion are not obsessing over food, diets, eating plans, or a scale. Our spirits and hearts are calling, begging for healing and nourishment, so we can expand and experience life.

Spiritual hunger is a calling from the heart. When we ignore this calling, we can find ourselves feeling that something undefinable is off. There may be a sense of longing rooted deep in our subconscious. When spiritual hunger is ignored, it is easy to try to fill the gaps with indulgent fast food and ignore what is begging for attention. It may be easier, but it will not fill the void in a lasting, meaningful, healing way.

I speak my personal truth here. This an area of my life in which I continue to be curious and meet myself in the inquiry. *What am I always chasing?* I ask myself. *What is there not enough of right now? What am I constantly trying to fill up on?*

This is spiritual hunger.

I don't mean to get all woo-woo about this—I am a practical, type-A, get-it-done kind of person. Even so, I recognize the importance of considering and honoring our spirit. Take time each day to be present. That means finding calm, quiet space to be with yourself in a state of peace. Listen for what your spirit has to say. Is there something it needs?

This is a simple, *free* practice you can tap in to, on your own terms, at your own will. It is a way to connect with yourself, yes, but also to connect with divine energy—God—who is doing work that we cannot possibly understand. Listen for your spirit calling.

So now it's your turn. Sit, close your eyes, take some deep breaths, and ask:

- *Who was I meant to be?*
- *What was I meant to do as my Best Diva?*
- *When I am not fighting myself with food and dieting, who do I envision myself as, trusting myself and having*

freedom, self-love, confidence, and newfound mental space?

- *Who am I?*

When I added bringing my awareness to my breathing, I discovered a feeling of centered calm and peace. I also discovered that I had a sense of calling and wisdom inside of me, one who had answers and who also had my back. I had just been so busy running my rat race of a life and chasing diets that the inner voice of wisdom had been crowded out.

I was learning to become one with my authentic self, allowing myself to feel that connection with my spirit and wisdom. Only after I experienced that feeling did I slowly begin healing my toxic relationship with food. With practice, I could feel and identify what my true non-food-related emotional and spiritual needs were at any given moment of any day. This allowed me to address those needs effectively, rather than reach for comfort foods or sugar. I felt liberated, inspired, and all of a sudden, capable.

What became clear to me is how much of my precious energy I had spent, for decades of my life, fighting diets, food, and myself. I was blind to my purpose in life based on the gifts I was given by God. I realized tearfully, in that moment, that I had left my free-spirited, people-loving, confident, happy, fun-loving little girl back in the fourth grade when I believed the facade of dieting.

I realize now that she is representative of my spiritual hunger. It was time for me to rescue her in my heart and free her as my authentic self who has a purpose to serve the world in empowering ways, starting with writing this book for you. I unleashed her once I honored my spiritual hunger, after I gave myself the mental space by ending my war with dieting.

I highly recommended you seek professional help if you feel trapped within yourself, especially if the trapped feeling is the result of past traumas, big and small. And, by the way, all traumas are valid and worthy of healing. It is okay to say you need help with feelings and emotions. It is okay to seek help to uncover what you've been stuffing away or avoiding.

We do not know what we do not know. Therapists, coaches, and counselors can help us find our way back to our hearts by helping us become open and curious. I was closed off from my heart and the world, guarding myself for so long. That was driving me to use food to escape myself.

With a trusted helper, it can feel safer—or at least tolerable—to open the door to what we've habitually shut down. It becomes possible to remain open and curious. We gain insight from counseling; we can discover a beacon for guided healing from within that we never knew how to find. This authenticity is paramount for ending our battle with food, body, and self.

Your Inner Queen Revealed

Your Queen emerges when you give her space, direction, and opportunity. Healing yourself from the inside out will satisfy your spiritual hunger and give you space to discover your Best Diva—who you were meant to be and what you were meant to do with your gifts from God. When you stand with her, you are at your best, doing your amazing thing in this world that was meant for you. You are your Best Diva Self.

And guess what else happens when you live your purposeful life?

Other people benefit. Anyone in your world, anyone who is touched by your work, your being, will be enriched by your full shining presence as you fulfill your life's purpose.

Your Queen is inside, ready to emerge as your Best Diva Self with the confidence to pursue what your spirit says you are meant to do.

CHAPTER FIVE

Preparing Your Path of Excellence

HARNESSING NEW HABITS

Chapter Four described the powerful mind-body-spirit trifecta as the foundational framework for healing our relationship with food, body, and self.

Your Path of Excellence represents the reliable, sustainable habits and tools that will support your diet-freedom journey toward your Best Diva Self on your terms.

Harnessing new habits to elevate an aspect of your life is a daunting task. Most of us begin with the best of intentions. Often, we do not detect the thing that takes over and prompts us to give up on ourselves.

I lived this way for decades when dieting. I'd write up my next diet plan and strategy on Sunday. I'd lay out all the rules and restrictions and then start on Monday.

This time it will work for me because . . .?

Well, I am not sure; I am simply going to do the same things I tried last time, but this time I will use more willpower.

Then, I'd falter. My inner voice would tell me once again: *I am a failure, and: There must be something wrong with me; I am weak.*

I'd start over with more rigid rules and hope for the best. I didn't understand what prevented me from harnessing new habits of eating for holistic nourishment. I gather many of you can relate in your own attempts to get a grip on your eating habits and make changes—to keep the promises you've made to yourself.

The Secret Cycle

James Clear, in his powerful book, *Atomic Habits*, describes a "Habit Loop" and four factors that work in sequence together to form a habit.

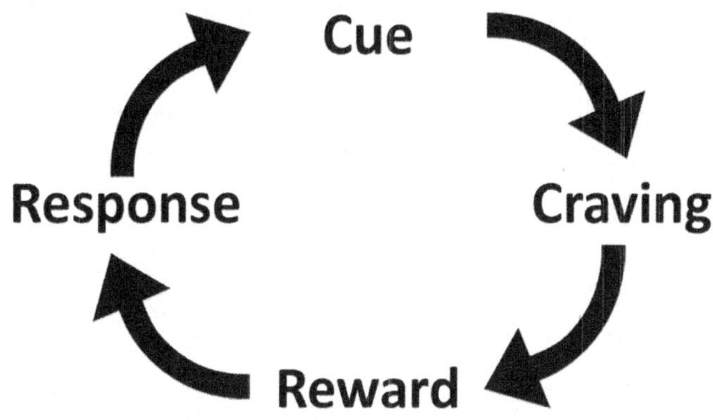

When we understand the four factors that build our habits, we can examine how the cycle applies to our attempts to find peace with food and body and perhaps discover what element is missing and keeping us stuck.

My own Habit Loop looked something like this:

Cue: I'd begin Monday with my promises in mind, follow through with my healthy eating and workout, and then, around 3:00 p.m., I'd be faced with something inconvenient or challenging, or I'd just forget myself and land in the low point of my day.

Craving: My emotions would become overpowering, and I'd feel helpless and in need of relief. I knew from my early conditioning that sugar makes me feel better—at least, in the moment—and brings relief to me immediately.

Reward: I'd go through the doughnut shop drive-thru like a mad woman and get a box of doughnut holes. I'd park my car, gobble them down within five minutes—often a dozen or more—and feel inner calm and relief washing over me from the dopamine-inducing sugar hit, the *legalized, socially acceptable drug*, as far as I'm concerned.

Response: Then the demoralizing inner chatter would follow. Suddenly, my promises to myself to eat the healthy foods I had planned for the day would become mentally distant. I'd yield to this triggering feeling and eat something sweet and chewy, giving up my healthy dinner plans in exchange for a binge on sweets. In this way, I felt like I was giving up on more than just my food plans; I was, in essence, giving up on myself.

After the response—bingeing on sweets, for example—there is a period of feeling disgusted and bloated, which can be toxic motivation to dust ourselves off, get up, and repeat our best intentions for the next day with some form of willpower that does not serve us. We all desire a Path of Excellence for food and body, one we can trust and sustain so we can get on with our lives, without the constant distractions and derailments.

Riding the Cycle

Instead of fighting or resisting this cycle, James Clear goes on to say our job is to embrace it. We must design strategies within the cycle to enhance our lives. In other words, we will always face the Cue—Craving—Reward—Response cycle.

Success comes when we allow ourselves to feel the stages in our cycle and learn to recognize them. The good news is you can learn to anticipate this loop. You can support yourself by *replacing and reframing* old thoughts and actions that have been keeping you stuck.

After the Cue, when the Craving hits, we can reframe our perception of the Reward, and our behavior in Response can be one of nurturance rather than self-sabotage.

Remember this cycle from an earlier chapter?

Thoughts → Feelings → Attitudes → Actions

We must first examine this as it relates to our inner relationship with our spirit and mind. This was such an epiphany to me—I had no idea how long I had been living with an inner disconnection that kept me running to food.

To change your perception and behavior involves elevating that Queen we talked about earlier and adopting an attitude of 100 percent responsibility for your decisions, thoughts, and actions. You do not need anyone else's approval or acceptance to make positive changes on your terms. You also do not need a scale or a deadline. *Whew!*

What you do need is to make some badass decisions that you are worthy enough to try for change, even when it means moving into initial discomfort. You need to be willing to move outside your *normal* behavior and to believe yourself worthy of the effort.

Remember your Top Three Values and your PPW that represents your motivational bull's eye. Without these front and center in your focus, life can take over and distract you, leaving you stuck and struggling and using food to cope and escape.

For what action will your future self thank your present self?

How can you accomplish keeping true to your PPW? Stop in that moment and immediately performing your Personal Inquiry.

Here are pivotal questions to consider at each phase of the cycle:

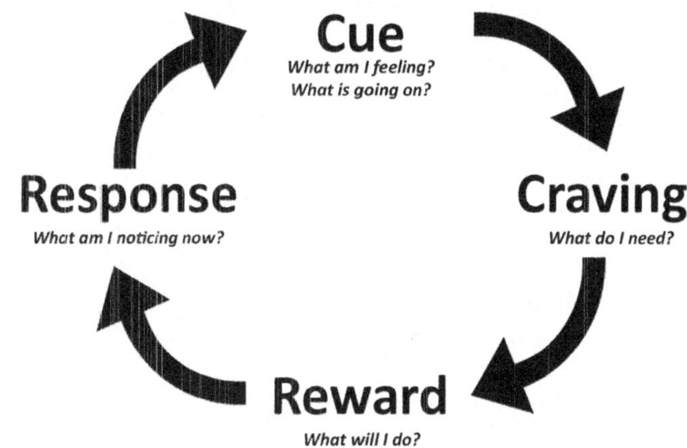

Friends, this is the power of *inquiry* and *mindset.* Most of us have been running on autopilot. We chase after our lives and ignore our feelings, true needs, and emotions. As a result, many of us have limited skills or understanding to just freakin' *stop* and have a personal conversation with ourselves to find out what the hell is going on inside and how to meet our needs in a nurturing way.

Think about how simple this sounds. If you are annoyed with me in this moment, *I get it!* We are having a breakthrough together. Here is your *truth*: your answers are inside your subconscious mind—inside your own head and heart. It is time to learn how to see past the noise and nonsense you have been tricked into believing. *You know* what is best.

Dieting is an illusion of how to solve a problem. The lie tells us we need to reshape our bodies into what we believe is the ultimate version of ourselves because we are *not enough* in our as-is state. When we submit to rules and restrictions with food, we are subconsciously choosing to ignore ourselves and our real needs—our real truths. We disconnect from our spirit, who knows us best, and connect to a battleground within. We sell out to what society tells us will work to *fix us*, and this always fails in the end.

Recognizing Snake Pits

Within the cycle, we inevitably encounter what I call *snake pits*. Snake pits are unplanned events or situations in which tempting foods you have chosen to avoid that day or challenging people show up. They are risks to our inner resolve to be mindful and to keep the promises we've made to ourselves. This is the reality and beauty of life. None of us exists in a land where there is 100 percent smooth sailing, a land where we have the free space and comfort to stay the course of excellence without any hazards—or snake pits—in the road.

Snake pits are situations in which you are faced with tempting foods that show up when you are within your 80 percent whole, natural foods choice of action. Your 20 percent that you save for planned occasions for savoring has been established and planned for future gratification. Snake pits are temptations and situations that challenge our perseverance on our path of excellence.

Here are examples:

- Office meetings where that tray of sugar-bastards is a regular staple
- Family celebrations where you are triggered by those opinionated bigmouths who send you for a mammoth slice of lasagna, or two, or three
- A bad day at work
- A fight with a spouse or friend
- Simply taking in the news

Expect and plan for snake pits. Two strategies for managing snake pits are doing your personal inquiry to connect with your feelings and what you really need, as well as drawing on your inner loving coach to guide you with supportive thoughts to help you adapt and adjust to challenging situations and stay true to your promises to yourself.

To discover your snake pits, ask yourself:

- *Who or what consistently derails me from my best attempts to choose healthy habit shifts?*
- *What situations or people make me feel vulnerable as hell?*

What we tell ourselves all day long is directly related to how closely we follow through on our designed Path of Excellence toward food, body, and self, as well as our ability to keep our promises to ourselves. To simplify, think of your thoughts as the fuel that directs your mind toward outcomes in your day that either keep you on your path or derail you.

Remember:

Thoughts→Feelings→Attitudes→Actions

Have you ever considered that your thoughts are holding you back from making sustainable changes in your life?

The thoughts rushing through our heads control the outcomes. Take the higher ground of *intention* to reboot your thoughts. Intentional programming—our new, purposeful thoughts—shape our feelings. The feelings become our attitudes, and our attitudes result in desired actions that elevate us in our relationship with food, body, and self.

Thought: *I have a big business meeting today at 3:00 p.m. There will be the usual junk foods there. I do not want to keep eating the junk that makes me feel horrible.*

Feeling: *I am nervous, but I really want to stay on plan with my promise. Can I do this?*

Attitude: *I am not going to worry about what others think because I am growing stronger each day in my relationship with me. I do not need or want those cookies because they do not love* *me back. I am going to stay true to my choices that elevate me, no matter what.*

Action: *I will bring my apple, nuts, and water bottle to the meeting. They will satisfy me and keep me on my Path of Excellence.*

Friends, this is not easy. This requires your willingness to consider the chatter and babble from your inner critic, the Wicked Witch, who has been holding you back.

She will continue to do her nasty work in your head if you allow her. Your inner loving coach, Glinda, is patiently supporting you from the sidelines. (Return to Chapter Three for a reminder about the common phrases these two voices utter.)

Consciously draw on Glinda's power and allow her to root for you all day long. You will probably notice a powerful shift in your attitude, the attitude that dictates your actions.

Constant inquiry, remember, means taking the time to *STOP!* and ask:

- *What am I feeling?*
- *What do I need?*
- *What will I do?*

Give yourself the gifts of *stopping* and *turning inward.* The ability to do this at any given moment is key to self-connection and self-inquiry. When we practice this, we grow in self-awareness, which provides space to understand our true needs in that moment. This can be the mega-tool to stop us from bolting to food and derailing our best attempts at developing healthy habits. This is being *mindful.*

Positive mental nutrition fuels our belief in ourselves, one day at a time. It helps us stay vigilant about inquiry throughout our day. Be aware and notice how you feel about yourself when you choose your planned snack over falling prey to a tempting sugar-bastard in a snake-pit moment. Recognizing this win is an empowering emotional investment in yourself that helps you build self-efficacy in riding the cycle and leveling up with a good habit.

CREATE YOUR STRONG FOUNDATION

Let's sit down together to map your Path of Excellence. On this journey you will travel in peace with yourself on your customized terms regarding food, body, self, and *your life.* Remember: How we eat is how we live. How we think is also how we live, by the way. Remember:

Thoughts → Feelings → Attitudes → Actions

Daily rituals provide a road map of small, customized, doable steps. These recurring steps ultimately make your goals attainable. Nothing will change unless you make a daily ritual that reinforces your goal—your PPW for your Best Diva Life.

The rubber meets the road here, friends.

Ask yourself these questions:

- *Do I only like the idea of designing my diet freedom road map, or am I willing to commit to intentional daily actions?*

- *Am I willing to try things that are uncomfortable in the beginning?*

- *Am I willing to follow through with my promised actions to myself even when I don't feel like it?*

- *Am I willing to give my best efforts one day at a time?*

- *Am I willing to do the work, to initiate my travel on the path toward achieving my Best Diva Life?*

After you establish with yourself that you're ready to commit, the next step is taking the time and effort to get *organized.* Your road map represents rituals that are meant to initiate the powerful tool of *changing your mindset.*

- What kind of person do you believe you are?
- What in your life do you believe you can change?

These questions help you to stay focused on your Top Three Values, PPW, and purposeful life. They help you direct your energy reserve toward the stuff that gets you where you want to go.

You have already discovered your three top values and your PPW. Those are huge steps that represent your motivational truths for what is important to you in your life—what you *really want* that is intrinsically valuable to *you*. Now it is time to lay out the rituals to jump on the road toward your Best Diva Life.

STEP FIVE: Tracking Your Path, Your 6 Ps, and Your Toolbox

PART A: Tracking Your Path to Excellence

Journaling is a powerful tool for rewriting our food story and breaking free from toxic dieting habits. I will admit I used to hate journaling because I was being told *what* to track in my journal according to the rules of the diet. I never really felt inspired by this until I decided to trash the typical standards of weight-loss journaling, which is often micromanaging food details and, of course, weighing yourself on the dreaded scale.

I basically gave the middle finger to traditional tracking for weight loss. Instead, I listened to what my inner wisdom *wanted* me to track. I began tracking things like my feelings, what I was grateful for that day, what success I had that day, and yes, my meals and snacks in a simple list. I also wrote down what I did for exercise.

A big key to my success was tracking what I did to calm down in the late afternoon instead of turning to sugar and carbs to get more energy. I developed a new habit of taking a ten-minute break in silence to reset, rejuvenate my mind, and relax. I was really stuck on that bad habit, and when I brought in some serious vigilance and awareness around *that particular thing*, I noticed that I had a history book of my healing journey in the making.

I now had a record of what was working for me that *replaced* using food to cope, numb, or escape. Momentum built like a chain, and I began to love this time with myself each day. The priceless takeaway here, that I did not even realize, is that I was training myself to become *mindful and self-aware*—two critical aspects of healing our relationship with food, body, and self.

Treat yourself to a fancy little journal that makes you feel special. Then track what the heck it is that *you want to keep track of* that will result in making positive changes. Examples include:

- Writing your feelings in the moment
- Three things you are grateful for
- A success from yesterday
- Three things you love about yourself
- Your meals and snacks
- How you moved your body/exercised
- One way you replaced a habit you're trying to shift

Sometimes it is helpful simply to write what happened that day and how you reacted in a nurturing way. Again, what you write must mean something to you and contribute to your awareness of progress and effort. Reading your progress and newfound relationship with self provides motivation. With this consistent habit, we begin to shed unwanted pounds naturally, and our looser-fitting clothes provide rewarding proof of our efforts.

PART B: The Six Ps of Planning

Motivational Speaker Brian Tracy has a famous saying: Proper planning prevents poor performance.

I have taken this quote and modified this as a tool for creating a Path of Excellence.

Proper Planning Promotes Powerful Personal Performance.

That is a graceful way of saying that we must plan for success, or we will fail.

Just as you would sit down to plan your route for a major road trip, you must, *must* take time to design your Path of Excellence with food, body, and self. The design comes from your commitment to implementing daily intentional rituals and strategies.

There is no *kinda sorta* approach to this. Without concrete, intentional decisions, you'll be stuck in the dreaming stage. Postponing your badass intentions has gone on long enough. Besides, your PPW is demanding your attention.

Here is where I dive into the Food and Body component of the trifecta of Best Diva Life, Mind, Body, and Spirit.

Whole, unprocessed foods are your staple.

Remember the 80/20 idea? Can you eat freakin' amazingly healthy foods that you like 80 percent of the time after your 14-Day Whole-Foods Cleanup we discussed in Chapter Four?

Now let's get back to the 80 percent. This involves intentional planning. Here is your simple weekly formula for success, using foods you love that love you back.

Plan + Shop + Prep = Success

Keep it simple.

Plan a few meals and snacks using foods that fit these criteria:

- You like these foods.
- They are convenient to prepare.
- They fit your lifestyle.
- They love you back by making you feel amazing from the inside out.

Yes, this works for take-out orders as well as eating in.

When deciding what to order or which groceries to buy:

- Use your common sense.

- Read nutrition labels.
- Keep it as close to nature as possible.
- Aim for low salt and low sugar.

I stick to a simple plan that satisfies me: A salad with protein, my choice of dressing on the side. I choose lean protein with no sauce as an entrée. I add a healthy starch and steamed veggies on the side. *Easy*. I've learned those foods make me *feel* great. Fettuccine alfredo makes me feel lousy.

Keep all triggery junk foods out of your house. No need for intruders who can take your power away on those bad days. We discussed planning for treats and indulgences on your terms for savoring. If we keep triggery foods in the house daily that are overly tempting to stop at a serving, we are setting ourselves up for disaster.

Pack and take your foods with you for best success. Again, *planning* is required here to navigate our junk-food-ridden society that will attempt to derail you at your weakest moments. If you have that apple and baggie of nuts with you, then you are supported.

Personal food planning is a must. People who enjoy abundant wellness and vitality prioritize meal and snack planning so that they have intentional control and focus over what goes into their bodies. You can do this too.

Plan meals and snacks that include whole, unprocessed foods. If it helps to repeat some of these foods, then do that.

I find success eating most of the same foods with a variety of healthy dinners each week.

What groceries will you need for one week?

Ideally, we shop for and cook our own foods. I recommend this and do so myself. However, if the thought of this tempts you to bolt for a pizza and give up, never fear! Use your good judgment and find local restaurants and takeout places that honor your whole, natural foods preference.

It is also a good idea to pack and take your foods with you, so you are prepared and not caught off guard, faced with foods that you have decided to avoid. I bring an apple, nuts, and water with me for emergencies. You can choose what whole-food go-to snack to bring based on your preference.

If you are serious about making healthy food shifts in your life, you will need to be very intentional about this. If it is a priority, you will find the time. That is the truth.

Will this go as planned all the time?

Heck no! And that is where the beauty of self-awareness comes in. You can make healthy choices on the fly *if*—again—*if* you are serious about keeping your promise to yourself to make healthy choices on your terms.

We do not need rules and micromanagement. We need common sense and a huge dose of mindful self-awareness each day. Making one loving choice at a time to honor our promise to ourselves is the way toward daily and enduring success.

PART C: Carry Your New Toolbox

Remember in Chapter One, I described how, as children, we take lessons from our early experiences?

Early experiences shape our beliefs about ourselves and the world. We put them in our subconscious *backpacks* and carry them with us for security. These beliefs often create limits in our minds, roadblocks and inner conflicting challenges that show up as eating challenges later.

My goal in this book is to bring clarity to what is missing from our focus when we somehow abandon our best intentions and give up on ourselves. The chosen diet, the food plan, the exercise plan, the rituals—I spent decades of my life playing mental Chutes & Ladders with diet attempts and failures, and I understand now that I was relying on that childhood backpack that did not serve my best self. The backpack needed to be emptied.

It's time to trade in your old backpack for a Toolbox of Treasures.

I still see life as a giant game of Chutes & Ladders, always moving forward with my best effort of the day. Sometimes I am climbing successfully and seamlessly, and sometimes I land on that space and am faced with a chute. Some unexpected curve ball sucker-punch drains my strength, attention, and energy and challenges me to my core.

This time, though, in my new game on my terms, I can land on that spot where I have a choice about whether I slide down again—escape with doughnuts and give up on myself—or stop, draw a tool from my treasure toolbox, and focus my attention and self-awareness mindset. Using the tool, I can look down that chute and say *nope, not today*, then put one foot in front of the other and progress along the game of life. I now know how to avoid self-sabotage in vulnerable moments.

Let's start building your toolbox of treasures. I believe that this, my friends, is a huge link that can save our lives as it relates to food, body, and self.

Remember, what we *think* becomes our *life*. How we do food is how we do life.

The Treasures Inside Your New Toolbox

If you have ever felt empowered to start a diet, you likely remember that fear of all the fast-food places, convenience stores, billboards, TV, advertisements, those middle aisles in the grocery stores they say to avoid, the dreaded checkout counters everywhere and anywhere that display junk food temptations that scream for attention and beg you to give up on your wellness goals and *eat them* for instant relief.

Friends, let's get real about this.

We simply cannot hide from or avoid them unless we want to go live in the desert.

Remember the suggestion of the 80/20 Idea and planning for splurges as 20 percent to avoid the trap of deprivation and restrictions?

I am asking you to honor and guard your 80 percent whole-food Path of Excellence with your toolbox. Impulsive eating takes a backseat when we remove restrictions and deprivations and instead, embrace that we *can* have treats and splurges. However, we are aware of how we feel when we eat certain things, and we understand the difference between planned savoring and impulsive sabotaging. This is giving our Inner Queen power and *adulting* with our food choices.

You may think: *I am powerless against my favorite junk foods.*

I get it! I used to fall impulsively hard for a Little Debbie snack cake or anything Hostess. This is not our fault, remember? Early conditioning with sugar and junk foods created this inner need and craving that we are now facing and slaying.

But it is still. So. Hard. I know.

What is the solution?

Allow me to introduce your newest super-tool—the dynamic duo of Special Glasses and INO!

Special glasses and INO are the two most important tools to draw on when dealing with any and all tempting situations with trigger foods. No need to run from them! No need to be afraid! You have badass Diva tools now. They will support you if you are vigilant and serious about them. They help you honor your 80 percent on the whole-foods Path of Excellence.

First, put on your special glasses. Of course, these are invisible glasses. Your special glasses provide strong truth, vigilance, and awareness of why you are choosing not to purchase or consume unhealthy foods. They contain the superpower of seeing beyond our temptation-driven society and staying on the narrow, unpopular road of honoring your 80 percent whole, natural, unprocessed food choices that keep you at your best.

Wearing special glasses, you learn to see tempting junk foods as objects instead of instant pleasures. Special glasses help you harness your inner Queen who reminds you that you make your healthy choices out of elevation, not deprivation. No need to fear the constant barrage of triggers when we wear our special glasses.

In addition to this super-tool, you have already fashioned rituals and goals for your life. You are working inside your badass Path of Excellence, where junk foods are simply not invited, not applicable, and do not fit in. Junk foods make us feel awful physically, mentally, and spiritually.

How?

They encourage us to jump on that chute and sliiiide back down to Start again, draining our precious self-trust and dignity.

With each clear decision, every successful situation in which we make that loving choice to say yes to our path and no to the junk, we build wellness and self-trust. We learn to recognize the feel of these better choices and register them as greater joys than that temporary hit of sugar-spurred dopamine.

***INO is short for* It's Not an Option**. This tool comes directly from Lisa Delaney's book, *Secrets of a Former Fat Girl*, in which she explains INO is a tool that gives you superpowers, like you're Captain Marvel or Wonder Woman. It is an invisible shield in your conscious mind that is ready and waiting for you to wield.

This tool helps you stay focused and on course with your 80 percent promise you are keeping to yourself in that triggering moment. INO is the tool that you immediately pull out to stop all whining, remembering, considering, feeling deprived—all that mental noise—before it starts. You see that pumpkin muffin at Dunkin when you are getting coffee, and *BAM!*

You think: *INO—it's not an option.*

Done. End of the thought. You did not even allow any former comfy-indulgent reference of that muffin. It is simply a thing, a noun sitting there. That is all. It's not an option to even think about that for a split second longer.

After you draw on INO, take on a reframing thought of *how great it feels* to follow through on your 80 percent promise with whole foods that love you back. Draw on your inner-loving-coach voice and tell yourself that you can enjoy that muffin on another day that honors your 20 percent for planned treats.

See how we navigate deprivation and use adulting skills instead?

Tell yourself how awesome you are for doing something radical, like not following society's sad foods anymore and how you are loving and protecting your boundaries by wearing your special glasses and using your INO in that moment. By doing so, you build confidence and self-trust.

Special glasses and INO work together so powerfully that cravings go away. These tools help us level up the adult voice within, who comes to our greater-good rescue when our inner child begins to kick and scream for junk foods. If we are implementing our 80/20 idea, we have planned our next occasion to indulge in treats and will savor them when the time comes. If our inner child begins kicking and screaming about a treat, and it is not within our 20 percent planned occasion, then the adult voice (in the form of INO and special glasses) takes over *fast* to quiet our child before the tantrum starts and to keep us on track with keeping our badass promises to ourselves that keep us on our path of excellence.

Cravings happen in our minds when we allow whiny thoughts of how sorry we feel for ourselves, how we *used to eat them*, or how *other people can*.

When you entertain those thoughts, they take over and pollute your mindset. The inner critic takes over, and you are vulnerable to caving and giving up on your goals.

If you begin to feel any sort of vulnerability coming from a trigger, whether visual or simply imagined, remember your special glasses and pull out your INO tool to *stop the thought in its tracks*. That's drawing on your inner loving coach, who reminds you of your priorities and where to focus next.

I have used special glasses and INO for years now, and I can honestly say that I rarely crave any of my old favorite junk foods. I face food triggers every day and am not fazed because I practice keeping my tools front and center in my mindset. I gave my daily rituals lots of time to take root in my mind, body, and spirit. Now I am a new version of myself that I trust.

And you can achieve this, too, with *effort, practice, and patience*.

Do I ever eat junk?

Yes! In fact, just last night I had birthday cake for my daughter's birthday. This day was planned as part of my 20 percent. I was able to savor a small piece of this cake with a newfound grace I never had.

And guess what? My stomach reminded me this morning why I do not eat sweets very often. I am grateful for this awareness because I no longer endure shame. I gave myself permission to enjoy that cake and savor it as my 20. Today, it's back to my 80 with grace and personal empowerment on my Path of Excellence that supports me. My special glasses are back on, and that cake has INO right in front of it in my mind.

Take back your power by ditching the scale. I found freedom to enjoy this no-endpoint, diet-free journey when I did *not* weigh myself. I found success in focusing on my daily habits that align with my path of excellence, not using the scale as a measure of success at all. I adopted the idea of *The Hanger Method*, in which I chose a pair of uncomfortably tight pants from my closet, hung them on a hanger in my bathroom where I had that visual goal in front of me each day, and tried them on each week as a motivational measure of success.

I felt a much greater reward when those pants finally slid on and zipped comfortably than a number on the scale, which I always believed should be lower—an example of a toxic limiting belief from past toxic dieting habits. This is powerful and positive motivational programming when we take back our power from those weigh-ins on the scale.

Find a Friend. Another powerful strategy is to find a friend in person or online who can journey alongside you—someone, or a group of others, who shares the common struggle with dieting and fighting oneself with food. It is pretty easy to find pals who share this, by the way. Choose companions who can offer confidential, nonjudgmental space and reciprocate with respect. Together, the accountability can be supercharged by the bond and supporting someone other than ourselves.

Keep It Super-Simple. The 5 Steps to Your Best Diva Life are meant to serve and support you for the long run, not stress or overwhelm you. Remember, we are talking about breaking free from dieting and insanity.

One of the main reasons diet programs lure us in is they sell us on their ways being best for us. We feel relieved that we don't have to figure it out for ourselves. We don't have to discover for ourselves the pathway for peace with food that supports our best health. It is easy to adopt dieting culture because we don't have to connect with ourselves. We don't have to create our own terms.

When you break free from dieting, you stop the clock. You block out the noise of the media. You sit with yourself, quiet the inner critic, harness the inner loving coach, and get real about a slow, sustainable approach for lasting results that are created by you, resonate with you, and work for you.

How do you keep it super-simple?

Start with one ritual, one small, positive change, to implement. Commit with intention to that one for a few weeks. Keep your promise to yourself, and don't break the chain. See what happens.

Then add another. Notice how keeping these promises to yourself is impacting you.

***Releasing* Stinkin' Thinkin', *aka* perfectionism.** Remember that we have identified that diets promote the kind of obedience that hijacks and toxifies our thinking. Diets also encourage us to equate judging our integrity and character as human beings to the degree that we are following our diet. We have been hard sold on this one. Add a splash of hardcore early conditioning to work hard and push forward, and it would make sense that we take on a belief system that is rooted in exaggerated expectations for perfection.

This unhelpful programming teaches us to believe that when we eat what is on plan and within points or macros, we are *good*. Go off-plan, even a little bit, for any—any—reason, exceeding points or macros, and we are *bad*. Worse than that—we are losers. We have failed.

In dieting, there is no wiggle room or gray area. It is black or white, win or lose, perfect or imperfect, success or fail. It is no wonder we are all off the rails, batshit crazier after every failed diet attempt to be *perfect* and live within this insanity.

Perfectionism can drive us to madness, becoming the tightrope between health and harm. I think of my love of aerobics and movement. While you might think these are healthful activities, because I was aiming for perfection, exercise was saving my life with one hand but killing me with the other.

I cultivated a two-headed monster when it came to perfectionism. I believed I had to follow the rules of my diet perfectly *and* I had to exercise excessively to achieve the perfect fitness-instructor role-model body to be respected and successful. Striving for these unrealistic expectations was exhausting and further fueled my binge eating refuge for escape.

I bought in to the identity and expectation of a fitness instructor to have the *perfect* body to be successful and respected. Everyone admired the skinny instructor or the one with the cut, chiseled body. I did manage to lose some of my high school pudginess by adding regular aerobics classes to my life, but my dieting strategies, rebellious binge eating, and ego intensified. My body was not skinny or chiseled, so I felt, on some level, second best. The fighter in me took over and so did my ego.

I tried throughout college and young adulthood to out-exercise my binge eating with intense aerobics classes. The restrictions I felt with dieting and striving to achieve an ideal body of a fitness instructor weighed heavily on my heart. The judgment was intense. Still, I would have sold my soul for the mistaken belief: *Once I get thinner, I will be happy and respected.* To me, fat meant failure, and skinny meant success.

Give up the stinkin' thinkin' and perfectionism!

Vow to never diet again, love all imperfections unapologetically, and become part of a movement to let your Path of Excellence lead you to the gray zone. This allows you to be comfortable with your best efforts in the ebb and flow of life, which is not linear, and where black-and-white, stinkin' thinkin', and perfectionism do not support you.

Get on with your Best Diva Life on your terms.

Will you have days when you ate a bit more than you planned, had an extra glass of wine, or finished someone's grilled cheese crust?

Hell, yes!

And guess what? That is living in the gray because you are recognizing this reality and knowing that wiggle room is part of common-sense self-care.

When we do not label ourselves with all-or-nothing thinking related to food, the drive to give up on ourselves or binge goes away. It no longer has a place because of how we are thinking about ourselves and tapping into our inner wisdom as our beacon, *not* a cookie-cutter, restricted food plan or macro tracker that we bought from someone else.

Conclusion

There is no fast track toward positive, sustainable, lasting changes. This book supports you to *change the way you live* and to change the way you see the world and the way you see yourself within it.

Your PPW and Best Diva Life are cultivated with loving patience, dedication to your promises, connecting to yourself through journaling, and *just* doing it, one day at a time. If you committed to X, Y, and Z, what version of you would emerge, with no end date—rather, a loving journey with no white-knuckling difficult rules. *Keep it super simple!*

Enjoy the day-by-day progress, knowing and trusting that you are in exactly the right place for you. I know it can be difficult to trust, particularly for recovering dieters. It can be tough to travel an uncharted road with lots of unkowns, but there is freedom and liberation in the unknown. It represents un-hijacked freedom of building self-trust, self-awareness, and self-confidence.

You learn with clear vision to see for yourself that your ways are best. One small successful step at a time builds your Path of Excellence. In this case, you will never need to diet again, nor will you ever need to recover from a binge that originated in your rebellion against a diet.

This has nothing to do with perfection. This has everything to do with finding happiness in your journey and taking small, daily steps to advance on your path.

Summary of the Trifecta

Dieting spreads toxic roots in our minds, bodies, and spirits. A powerful shift occurs when we discover how dieting is an anti-solution to weight loss and our best selves. The road to reclaiming one's free spirit is available to everyone. In the previous chapters, I have outlined the solutions to losing weight and finding your Best Diva Self by means of a healing trifecta of mind, body, and spirit. Here is a summary:

1. **Mind**. Face and heal old wounds with openness and curiosity. Develop your inner loving coach to help you build powerful self-awareness, which provides loving, compassionate space to process your feelings and to tend your true needs at all times. This is the pathway to end emotional eating challenges.

Remember the three questions:

What am I feeling?
What do I need?
What will I do right now?

2. **Body**. Choose unprocessed whole foods you enjoy that serve your best physical and mental health. Associate food with self-care and pleasure that can

be sustained for a lifetime by striving for quality and reasonable quantity. Form a new relationship with food that demonstrates your desire for self-care and savoring, not self-sabotage. Understand choosing to move your body brings energy and vitality. Movement keeps your body physically strong and functional for life.

3. **Spirit**. Connect with your inner wisdom and consciousness that lives in your heart and mind. This is God, who is our ultimate healer. Our spirit guides us toward meeting our needs in a loving, compassionate way and ends the inner battle. With this newfound freedom, mental space, and self-trust, you elevate your inner Queen with newfound confidence to unleash your purpose in life. *Look out, world, here comes your Best Diva!*

Friends, mind-body-spirit balance is the ticket to smart healing from the destruction debacle that we have created with dieting. Remember: One day at a time, with loving perseverance and commitment, with no end point, are the keys to weight loss success without ever dieting again. You are elevating your sensible, mature, inner Queen and getting real about healing.

We are all worthy of giving ourselves a chance to taste the truth and the gift of wellness and best health. We are all capable of doing the work to experience this. Once you *taste* what this is for you, the rest is unlimited, and your dieting days will be a thing of the past.

The gift to yourself for honoring and living within your personally designed Path of Excellence is your Best Diva Self, unleashed with confidence and strength. This is *you*, claiming your place in this world. Here is where you rewrite your story.

You may discover that when you have newfound mental space, you reclaim who you were born to be. The world needs you at your best to serve your purpose as you were meant to do, authentically and unapologetically.

I cannot wait to see who you discover yourself to be in this freedom. The world needs you to serve your purpose and cannot wait anymore behind some nonsensical war with food and a diet that keeps you hijacked and distracted from your true self. It's just you and me in this journey called *life* and *healing*.

I am on your team and rooting for you, as together we walk the journey down our Path of Excellence to discover the badass selves we are deep down inside.

Let's get out there and do what we are meant to do with passion and power and *never* diet again. We know better.

ONWARD!

Summary of the 5 Steps to Become Your Best Diet-Free Diva

STEP ONE: Discover and write your food story.

STEP TWO: Identify your Top Three Values and write your Personal Powerful Why (PPW).

STEP THREE: Commit to daily personal inquiry and master your self-awareness.

STEP FOUR: Perform your 14-Day Whole-Foods Cleanup Experiment.

STEP FIVE: Commit to daily journaling for tracking your Path of Excellence; define and implement your 6 Ps, and carry your new toolbox.

Next Steps

Making the decision to turn away from diets and to trust yourself to find your best self and freedom for food and body is no easy task, especially when we are constantly barraged with the media attempting to lure us into believing that diets are the way.

Congratulations for your courage in considering a fresh perspective in which you can shift out of dieting drama and into finding your own terms for elevating your best health. I admire your willingness to consider that you have your own answers right in front of you. With a little curiosity and an inquiry, you could discover your unique secret to releasing the shackles of fighting food and its associated emotional eating challenges.

Liberation and transformation can be yours for the taking. The first steps are the hardest. I tried to go it alone for decades; I hid in my shame, and I failed miserably. My heart ached. My healing happened only when I found support with wonderful coaches and a community of loving, like-minded friends who shared my struggles. I really thought that no one else had my problem regarding food. I am so happy that I found out I was so wrong.

You are worthy of being heard in your struggle without judgment or criticism. I would be honored to hear your story and support you with empathy, grace, and loving guidance to help you find *your* unique pathway of healing by programming the 5 Steps toward dieting freedom and Best Diva Self presented in this book.

I would be honored to give you the open space that you deserve right now, and help you take first your step, writing your Food Story. To schedule your free sixty-minute confidential connection, reach out to me, and I will guide you through the additional steps and the Powerful Trifecta to help you design your Path of Excellence toward your Best Diva Self!

Contact: tracy@theholisticdivas.com

Website: theholisticdivas.com

Meanwhile, as a gift to you, my beloved reader, click this link to get your very own template for brainstorming your 5 Steps for Dieting Freedom, and begin your journey toward harnessing your Best Diva Self:

theholisticdivas.com/dietfreediva

This is your first empowering action toward breaking free of the shackles of dieting and moving onward to create your sustainable, result-oriented Path of Excellence.

References

Certification Program:

Institute for the Psychology of Eating. Marc David, founder.

Books:

Delaney, Lisa. *Secrets of a Former Fat Girl.* The Penguin Group. 2007.

Moss, Michael. *Salt, Sugar, Fat.* Random House. 2013.

Simon, Julie M. *The Emotional Eater's Repair Manual.* New World Library. 2012.

Simon, Julie M. *When Food is Comfort.* New World Library. 2018.

About the Author

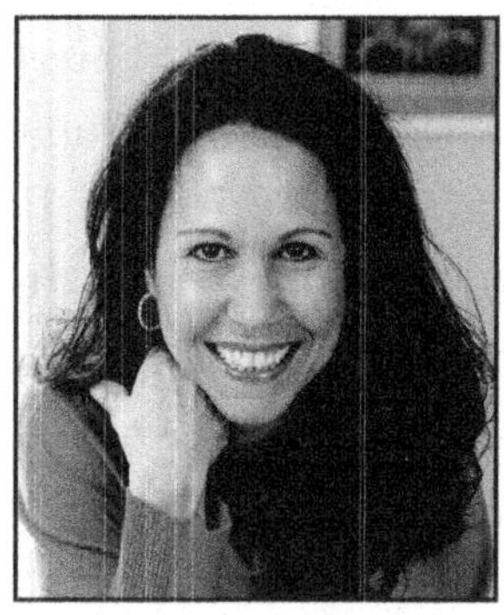

Tracy L. Desjardins is a Certified International Health Coach (IAHC), a Mind Body Eating Coach (Institute for the Psychology of Eating), and a Certified Personal Trainer and Group Fitness Instructor (American Council on Exercise). Tracy has shifted her thirty-plus-year fitness career into coaching holistic wellness for women. Tracy specializes in emotional eating recovery and healing from the damage of dieting, restricting, and binge eating. Tracy is especially passionate about this healing after spending decades of her life battling her own challenges with food, body, and self.

Tracy dedicates her coaching to helping other women find freedom from the shackles of dieting, emotional binge eating, and excessive exercising to find peace with food, body, and self *on their terms*. Her holistic approach provides a pathway for women to liberate themselves from restrictive, toxic, diet programming. It guides them to find their own sustainable Path of Excellence with food, body, and self so women can live their Best Diva Lives.

Tracy is based on the Eastern Shore of Maryland with her husband, Gary. They have two adult children, Emily and Jackson. Originally from western Pennsylvania, Tracy attended Saint Vincent College in Latrobe, Pennsylvania, and has a Bachelor of Arts in Business Administration.